Unleash Your Inner Health!

Unleash Your Inner Health!

Harness Your Body's Desire to be Healthy & Fit in 21 Days!

Copyright 2017

Please follow Dr. Blair on social media and visit his website often for updates and inspiring stories of healing.

Dr. Blair is available for media appearances and speaking engagements through his website

JeffBlair.org

Dr. Jeffrey Blair PhD

Table of Contents

Forward

by
Ricky Williams
Heisman Trophy winner / 11 Year NFL star / Celebrity
Apprentice star (NBC) / Yoga Master / Ayurvedic Healer /
Cranial Sacral Practitioner

When I played professional football, I spent roughly six months of every year pounding my body and brain into the equivalent of several Mack trucks. I took on abuse most humans would run from— but I ran toward it, at award-winning speed. During that time, I had a diet of everything from donuts and prescription meds, to media persecution for the opposite—fresh air, yoga, and cannabis. There were years of sporadic regimens that spiraled my weight and stress levels, up and down. If anyone knows about the worse a body can take, I'd say it was me.

However, there was another six months out of that year that I would do the opposite, following a course of nurturing that included research, scholarship through various academic and vocational courses, trips around the world, and meetings with various healers. I attribute that time to what saved me from conditions that have sadly befallen many former athletes. Tests that should have shown permanent damage from directly applied abuses, instead showed what some would consider a miracle.

It doesn't take a miracle to achieve balanced health (even when your profession requires you do the opposite). When I discovered the ideas and guidelines presented by Dr. Jeffrey Blair I realized how pertinent they would be for this particular era. There is more information on health and wellness available today, at the click of a button, than has ever been, yet there has never been a greater health crisis. People spend all twelve months abusing themselves both willfully and inadvertently, despite the wealth of information. What Dr. Blair offers is first, mental dieting; or training the mind for fitness—which is every bit like any preconditioning that an athlete might receive. Then he adds specific researched remedies which many, including myself, have found to be nutritional sparks to ignite a better way to live, not just eat.

After learning about herbs, he became intrigued with how they can help with stress. During a visit to Austin, Texas, where I was living at the time, we met and spoke at length about everything from yoga and the alleviation of stress, to the medicinal aspects of cannabis. After our talk, I came to the agreement that an inability to manage stress leads to many illnesses of the mind, body, and spirit. Therefore, it's essential we reconsider alternatives like herbs and natural plants etc. because our current model isn't working. That's what I most appreciate about the direction Dr. Blair's, *"Unleash Your Inner Health"* takes us in. Whether he is talking about dieting, running, identifying and reducing stress—or the holistic benefits of herbs you may be overlooking—every chapter is a map towards your own personal miracle. – *Ricky Williams*

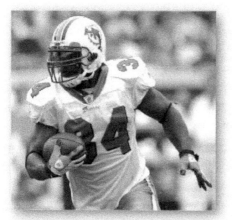 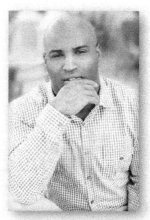

Ricky Williams playing for the Miami Dolphins…and today

From Dr. Blair's Blog

How Silkworm Vomit Can Save Your Life!

Okay, I know this sounds gross but hear me out on this one. Silkworms produce an enzyme called serrapeptase that just might save your life. Serrapeptase comes from the digestive system of the silkworm, when the silkworm regurgitates (vomits) serrapeptase to break free from its cocoon. Serrapeptase is a proteolytic enzyme. This means that it breaks down protein into smaller components (peptides and amino acids) that the body can easily use. Scientists in India have studied the enzyme serrapeptase to see how it could be used in the human body.

They proved that serrapeptase is a very powerful anti-fibrotic enzyme! And several more research studies came to the same conclusion. Anti-fibrotic enzymes break down a protein called fibrin that can be very damaging when it builds up in the body. Fibrin build up is called fibrosis and can result in abnormal thickening or scarring of fibrous connective tissue.

Examples of Conditions Causes by Fibrosis:

- **Plaque buildup on the arterial walls (atherosclerosis)**
- **Fibrocystic breast disease**
- **Uterine fibroid tumors**
- **Scarring after injury**
- **Scarring after surgery**
- **Cystic Fibrosis; affecting the exocrine glands (secreting glands; mucus, hormones, etc.) of the lungs, liver, pancreas, and intestines.**
- **Blood clots; due to the fibrin in blood**

Luckily, you don't have to catch a silkworm to get its serrapeptase. It is available in capsule form and taken on an empty stomach can increase circulation and prevent dangerous blood clots.

Introduction

There is a health crisis in our country. The obesity rate continues to climb despite spending millions of dollars every year on the latest fad diet. More people are in pain now than ever before despite spending trillions of dollars on pain medications. Heart disease and cancer continue to be the leading causes of death despite all the money spent on research and medicine. Type 2 diabetes rates are at an all-time high and continue to grow. People are tired and stressed in a fast-paced society that turns to caffeine to get through each day and modern medicine has been unable to slow down any of these trends.

I have spent over 25 years studying nutrition and herbal medicine. I have scoured 3000 years of research and traditional use of herbs from villages around the world. My purpose in writing this book is simply to invoke thought. As I am not a Medical Doctor I cannot diagnose or treat disease. This book is not intended to be medical advice and I would never advise anyone to disregard their doctor's advice. I am simply inviting you to open your minds and take control of your own health by doing research and making an informed decision.

Dietary supplements are big business. In the Unites States, sales totaled over $37 billion in 2016. According to estimates by the National Institutes of Health more than one-third of all Americans take some form of dietary supplement in any given month. Among seniors over the age of 71, 48 % of women and 43% of men use them. Other estimates place the total number of supplement users in the U.S. as high as 69%.

Vitamins, minerals and herbal supplements have a tremendously safe track record, yet they are often singled out as being potentially dangerous by government agencies like the U.S. Food and Drug Administration (FDA) and others. For many years now, an organized campaign has been waged against supplements, with the aim of regulating them as drugs rather than food, as is currently the case.

Even when taken as prescribed, drugs kill an estimated 106,000 Americans each year and that's using decades-old data. Today people use more drugs, so the death toll could be much higher. The same cannot be said for nutritional supplements. Data provided in a 2012 report by the U.K.-based Alliance for Natural Health International, showed that adverse reactions to pharmaceutical drugs are 62,000 times more likely to kill you than food supplements.

Orthomolecular Medicine News Service reported "There were no deaths whatsoever from vitamins in the year 2014. The 32nd annual report from the American Association of Poison Control Centers shows no deaths from multiple vitamins. And, there were no deaths whatsoever from vitamin A, niacin, vitamin B-6, any other B-vitamin. There were no deaths from vitamin C, vitamin D, vitamin E, or from any vitamin at all."

It can be conclusively said about nutritional supplements that they may be the safest category for any consumable product yet the pharmaceutical and medical establishment are waging war on the supplement industry.

I will discuss my thoughts on why we are in a health crisis as well as research into the roles that proper nutrition and herbs play in maintaining and regaining health. Health is a journey that is never too late to begin! Our bodies were designed with a remarkable ability to heal and stay healthy if given the right tools. I will teach you that by redefining yourself and strengthening your mental attitude, making some easy dietary changes, and taking proven, safe nutritional supplements you can Unleash Your Inner Health!

Transform Your Body in 21 Days!

In order for you to achieve optimum health, lose weight, reduce disease, and live a fit & healthy life, you must realize that it will take some effort. A healthy & fit body begins between the ears and the mind plays a huge role in our health. In this book I will lay out a plan to help you lose weight permanently while reducing the risks of heart disease, diabetes, and cancer. I will discuss natural ways to reduce pain, lower blood pressure, balance blood sugar, sleep better, increase youthful energy, improve mood, and much more! This plan does not start with a new diet, supplement, or exercise program. It starts with changing the way you think about yourself by re-defining "who" you are and by changing daily habits.

How often have you or someone else said *"I should lose weight"*? This happens all the time and is one reason that most diets fail in the long term. It is necessary to change the way you think to insure success. You'll rarely achieve what you **"should"** do, but you have a much better chance at achieving what you **"must"** do! In other words, if you decide that you **must** lose weight you'll have greater success. You will have to decide that you must lose weight and regain your health before it can happen! This is accomplished by changing your daily habits and that takes at least 21 days of repetition.

In the 1950's, a plastic surgeon named Maxwell Maltz determined that it takes at least 21 days to form a habit. He determined this by observing his patients recoveries from surgeries as well as observing changes in his personal life and published his theory in 1960. Then, in a 2009 study published in The European Journal of Social Psychiatry, researchers tested 96 people and determined it takes an average of 66 days to form a new habit. My feeling is that whether it takes 21 days or 66 days, you must begin with day 1!

If you will follow my outline for Unleashing Your Inner Health for at least 21 days you will be well on your way to making the mental changes necessary to transform your body and your life! It may take longer than 21 days for some but the destination is well worth the journey. Re-define yourself as someone that **must** get up and go exercise every day. Re-define yourself as someone that **must** reduce the sugar in your diet. Re-define yourself as someone that **must** spend time laughing, praying, meditating, and in motivation every day. Re-define yourself as someone that **must** spend time doing research on health conditions so that you can make an informed decision about your healthcare. If you do these "**musts**" every day for at least 21 days you will Unleash Your Inner Health. You are who you <u>think</u> you are!

From Dr. Blair's Blog

Nostradamus & the History of Herbal Medicine

The use of plants as medicine dates back to the beginning of time. There is written word of the use of herbs in the book of Genesis in the Bible. The Egyptians and Chinese wrote of herbal remedies several thousand years ago and the Greek physician Hippocrates wrote about herbal treatments around 400 B.C.

As an herbal medicine historian I am passionate about learning all I can about the history of using plants as medicine. Several years ago I learned about an herbal healer from France in the 1500's that is much more known for predicting the future. His name is Michel de Nostredame, or Nostradamus. Nostradamus is well known for writing his quatrains of predictions but few know that he was also an apothecary in 16th century France. An apothecary was a dispenser of medicine, and some scholars believe he went to medical school and became a physician. The most impressive accomplishment of Nostradamus was not a prediction he made but his role in ending the plague of the 1500's.

It was Nostradamus that came up with the "unique" idea that the doctors of the time should wash their hands before surgery and that human waste should be washed from the streets. He also invented a medicine to strengthen the immune systems of the afflicted which consisted of rose hips (vitamin C).

Today, the World Health Organization estimates that 80% of the world's population still relies on plant medicines and it's easy to see why. The facts are that up to 150,000 people die each year from prescription drug side effects (JAMA), while no one died from herbal or nutritional supplements (CDC). Plant medicines are safe and effective with a history that spans over 8,000 years.

1

Blindly Follow

We are living in a sea of information, yet drowning in ignorance! We have never lived in a time where so much information is at our fingertips. We can simply "Google" any topic we want and get hundreds and thousands of references to look up. So why is it that so many people don't take full advantage of this amazing time of information overload, especially when it comes to their health?

Let me begin by stating up front that I am not "anti-doctor"! Nor am I against prescription drugs. I believe that there is a place for both but that "modern" medicine has let us down. Modern medicine has done some wonderful things to keep people healthy. People are living longer thanks to certain vaccines, medicines, and surgeries. 100 years ago the leading cause of death was infection, so the discovery of antibiotics was groundbreaking science that has prolonged millions of lives. Open-heart surgeries and organ transplants are examples of modern medicine at its finest and have saved many lives, and if I am ever in a car accident or have a heart attack (or other medical emergency) please take me to an emergency room trauma center where I feel confident they can save me!

So, modern medicine has accomplished many great things and it has a place, but it has also failed us miserably in many areas. We have been misled by the medical establishment, the media, and our government for many years about health. There are campaigns costing millions of dollars every year against the use of natural remedies and nutritional supplements. We are constantly being told that it is too risky to trust our health to "unproven" herbs and vitamins, and that we should trust "approved" pharmaceuticals. In a time of information overload at our fingertips it is appropriate for us to do our own research and take control of our health. Why must we blindly follow what the medical establishment tells us without doing our own research? After all, it is our body and health at stake and modern medicine has had many failures. Here is a fun experiment although my wife turns the channel now and won't let me do this anymore: next time a commercial comes on TV for a prescription drug, take the time to actually listen to the side effects. You won't have to wait very long because every 3rd or 4th commercial is pushing a drug on us! While the lady with the pleasant voice is reading all the horrible side effects, many including increased risk of suicide, heart disease, cancer, and sudden death, simply ask yourself "is the reward worth the risk"?

According to The Journal of the American Medical Association (JAMA), side effects from properly prescribed pharmaceutical drugs are responsible for well over 106,000 deaths each year. While people are dying following the advice of the medical establishment we are constantly being told to continue just blindly following their recommendations while avoiding addressing any underlying cause or treatment with natural remedies. There are many time-tested herbal remedies that have a remarkable history of healing being suppressed by modern medicine. You see, medicine is a multi-trillion dollar business and there is no profit in health. I'm not talking about individual doctors or pharmacists trying to keep people sick for profit! **I do believe that most doctors and practitioners are truly interested in people being healthy**. I am talking about the system here…a system that trains physicians to prescribe dangerous drugs to treat symptoms while ignoring underlying nutrition deficiencies and lifestyles. The "system" is rigged for massive profit and has no interest in promoting true health. I spoke with a recent graduate of medical school who told me that he had learned nothing about nutrition. How can doctors be in charge of our health when they're not taught about how to keep the body healthy? The answer is simple…we must be in charge of our own health!

Three of the largest failures of modern healthcare are pain management, ADHD, and cholesterol. I will briefly discuss why I think we have been misled and failed by modern medicine.

Chronic Pain

According to The National Center for Health Statistics over 76 million people suffer with daily, chronic pain. That's more than suffer from diabetes, cancer, and heart disease combined! The top reported chronic pain is back, neck, and migraine. The most widely used pain killers are non-steroidal anti-inflammatory drugs (NSAIDS) including over-the-counter Ibuprofen, Naproxen, and aspirin. NSAIDS are responsible for over 100,000 hospitalizations and 15,000 deaths each year. There are many possible side effects of taking NSAIDS including gastrointestinal bleeding, allergic reaction, hearing loss, and up to a 60% increase in risk of heart disease! On September 30, 2004 the FDA approved prescription NSAID Vioxx was pulled from the market after 139,000 reported heart attacks and 60,000 deaths! Other prescription NSAIDS have been pulled and many at the FDA say that all prescription NSAIDS are associated with increased risk of heart attack.

Doctors now are all too often prescribing powerful opioid pain killers. The United States is in the midst of an opioid overdose epidemic. According to The National Center for Health Stats over 28,000 people died last year from opioid use, including one of the greatest musical geniuses of our time…Prince. It is estimated that 91 people die daily from opioid use and it doesn't have to continue. There are natural pain relievers with a proven track record of safety and efficacy that are being ignored by the medical establishment because they profit more by pushing their drugs! I will discuss several of these, including cannabis, in later chapters. Cannabis has a proven ability and has been used as a natural pain killer for thousands of years yet our government suppresses it and keeps it illegal. It is classified as a schedule 1 drug meaning it has NO medicinal value yet the Department of Health and Human Services holds a patent (#6630507) stating that cannabinoids (from cannabis) are useful in the treatment of inflammatory disease (pain relief), auto-immune disease, and neurological disease. I will discuss this in greater detail later but for now it's appropriate to ask the question… "How can the government say that cannabis is a dangerous drug with no medicinal value while holding a patent saying that it DOES have medicinal value"? To me, the answer is simple. Of course they know cannabis is a powerful medicine but because it is a natural plant found in nature it cannot be sold as a prescription therefore there is no money to be made by big pharma. They go to great lengths to keep this natural medicine from us so they can continue profiting by selling dangerous, deadly drugs for trillions of dollars. And, according to The Substance Abuse and Mental Health Services Administration there has never been a death recorded from the use of cannabis! NEVER! Not ONE! And we continue to blindly follow…

Cholesterol Hoax

The next big failure (scam) has been the war on cholesterol. Cholesterol is one of the most important substances found in our body. In fact, we cannot live without it! It is a necessary component of every human cell and is the foundation of all hormones. 25% of cholesterol is found in the brain because it cannot function properly without it. Cholesterol is made in the liver naturally and is needed to make another vital (yet grossly deficient) nutrient vitamin D (really a hormone). I'll devote an entire chapter later to the importance of vitamin D as it is truly a remarkable nutrient that we cannot live without. It is easy to see though why over 85% of Americans are deficient in this life-giving vitamin… for many years we have been told that the sun and cholesterol are deadly killers and both must be avoided. Well, our body converts cholesterol into vitamin D in the presence of sunlight and we've been told to avoid the two things vital to its production. And we blindly follow...

The cholesterol myth starts back in 1953 when biologist Ancel Keys proposed the theory that fat in the diet caused heart disease. He studied the fat intake of people in seven countries (The Seven Countries Study) and found that there was a link between fat consumption and heart disease. The study was flawed however as he did not take into account the amount of sugar being consumed as well. Many studies since then have proven Keys wrong in his analysis and Keys himself in 1997 said "There is no connection between cholesterol in food and cholesterol in blood, and we've known this all along". A British doctor named John Yudkin did a more thorough investigation and determined that sugar intake was a larger contributor to heart disease than fat. Another British doctor named Malcolm Kendrick used Keys data and proved that those that ate the **most** fat and cholesterol had **lower** risk of heart disease (M Kendrick The Great Cholesterol Con). So as you can see, Keys theory was questioned and debunked early on and there have been many more studies since that have linked sugar intake to heart disease and not fat or cholesterol.

According to Dr Joseph Mercola *"Your total cholesterol level is NOT a great indicator of your heart disease risk. Cholesterol could easily be described as the smoking gun of the last two decades. It's been responsible for demonizing entire categories of foods (like eggs and saturated fats) and blamed for just about every case of heart disease in the last 20 years".*

The cholesterol guidelines and recommendations keep getting lower and lower despite evidence that low cholesterol does not prevent heart disease and can actually be dangerous. In order to achieve these outrageous and dangerously low numbers, you typically need to take multiple cholesterol-lowering drugs. So the guidelines instantly increased the market for these dangerous drugs. Now, with testing children's cholesterol levels, they're increasing their market even more, all for profit over health concerns.

Dr. Ron Rosedale MD says *"Cholesterol is your friend, not your enemy"*

"Before we continue, I really would like you to get your mind around this concept. In the United States, the idea that cholesterol is evil is very much engrained in most people's minds. But this is a very harmful myth that needs to be put to rest right now. First and foremost, cholesterol is a vital component of every cell membrane on Earth. In other words, there is no life on Earth that can live without cholesterol. That will automatically tell you that, in and of itself, it cannot be evil. In fact, it is one of our best friends. We would not be here without it. No wonder lowering cholesterol too much increases one's risk of dying. Cholesterol is also a precursor to all of the steroid hormones. You cannot make estrogen, testosterone, cortisone, and a host of other vital hormones without cholesterol."

A review of research published in BMJ Open Journal conducted at Lund University in Sweden and the University of Ireland found that 92% of people with a high cholesterol level lived longer. Dr. Sherif Sultan of the study said *"cholesterol is one of the most vital molecules in the body and prevents infection, cancer, muscle pain, and many other conditions"* and that *"The benefits of statin treatment have been greatly exaggerated".*

Statin drugs are dangerous and can cause severe muscle pains, kidney failure, suicidal thoughts, depression, depletion of CoQ10, and Alzheimer's disease. They have also been proven ineffective. Pfizer's Lipitor is the most prescribed cholesterol medication in the world and has been prescribed to more than 26 million Americans. According to Lipitor's own Web site, Lipitor is clinically proven to lower bad cholesterol 39-60 percent, depending on the dose. Sounds effective but BusinessWeek actually did an excellent story on this very topic and they found the real numbers right on Pfizer's own newspaper ad for Lipitor.

At first glance, the ad boasts that Lipitor reduces heart attacks by 36 percent. But there is an asterisk. And when you follow the asterisk, you find the following in much smaller type: "That means in a large clinical study, 3% of patients taking a sugar pill or placebo had a heart attack compared to 2% of patients taking Lipitor."

What this means is that for every 100 people who took the drug over 3.3 years, three people on placebos, and two people on Lipitor, had heart attacks. That means that taking Lipitor resulted in just one fewer heart attack per 100 people. One hundred people have to take Lipitor for more than three years to prevent one heart attack. And the other 99 people, well, they've just dished out hundreds of dollars and increased their risk of a multitude of side effects for nothing. So you can see how the true effectiveness of cholesterol drugs like Lipitor is hidden behind a smokescreen. In 2008 it was discovered that two other statin drugs (Zetia and Zocor) actually made plaque buildup WORSE.

As always, I am not advising that you go against your doctor's advice. My intentions are only to educate and encourage people to seek out information to make an informed decision about their health.

Attention Deficit Hyper-Activity Disorder

This is the failure that bothers me the most because it involved our children. All too often kids are being "diagnosed" with ADHD and prescribed a powerful stimulant. Let's look at it this way: If I go down to the street corner where drug dealers hang out and buy cocaine or methamphetamine from a dealer, I'm breaking the law by buying an illegal, dangerous drug! But, if my 12 year old child has trouble paying attention or is a little hyper the pediatrician can sell us that same drug as medicine! That's right, the drugs that the doctor prescribes for ADHD is the same drug the criminal dealer is pushing on the street! Both are amphetamines listed as a schedule 2 drug. I think it is **outrageous** that children today are being given these elicit harmful drugs in an attempt to calm them down.

I have interviewed many parents and children about their experiences with an ADHD diagnoses and it always amazes me that for the most part the doctor never even attempts to address the underlying

cause of the attention issue or hyperactivity! This to me is criminal as it is putting our children at great risk of addiction and health issues and was amazed at the number of adult addicts had been prescribed an ADHD medication as a child. Additionally, in college, I observed cocaine addicted monkeys given ADHD prescribed amphetamines not be able to tell the difference between the cocaine and the prescription. And modern medicine feels that it's necessary to drug our youth with these powerful stimulants without attempting to address and correct the underlying causes.

Let's look at a pretty typical day in the life of a child:

- Eat a sugar-filled breakfast
- Go to school with spiked blood-sugar causing excitability and hyperactivity
- A few hours later, spiked blood-sugar crashes causing attention issues
- Go to lunch (or vending machine) and eat high carb meal with sugar-filled drink
- Go back to class with spiked blood-sugar (excitability & hyperactivity)
- Sugar crash (fidgeting & Attention issues)
- Repeat…

This is the typical behavior that gets many children labeled ADHD and prescribed these cocaine-like drugs to help focus when needed and calm them down when needed. When I was a kid this is how we acted and it was labeled "normal".

I've been on a crusade against ADHD "diagnoses" and drugs for over 20 years and have seen many children get off of and/or avoid taking these drugs simply by addressing the underlying cause. The culprit in most cases is dietary and can easily be fixed. In the sample above notice that the common ingredient in each meal was sugar. Sugar and starchy carbs raise blood-sugar levels contributing to ADHD symptoms as well as obesity and diabetes. I will teach you in a later chapter that it is possible to achieve great health by changing the way you think. In this case, parents need to change their dietary routines and habits for the health of their children. Another major cause of ADHD symptoms is magnesium deficiency. 85% of adults are deficient in magnesium and even more children are. Magnesium is one of the most important minerals, necessary for proper heartbeat, muscle function, and cognitive function, and is grossly deficient from kids' diets! If your diet contains white sugar, white bread, white rice or other processed foods – you are deficient in magnesium. Let's look at "symptoms" of ADHD:

- Impaired communication
- Social difficulties
- Restlessness
- Tantrums
- Can't keep still, constant body rocking
- Noise sensitivity
- Poor attention span, poor concentration
- Irritability, aggressiveness

If you go to the doctor with any or several of these symptoms you are more likely than not going to walk out with a prescription for a dangerous drug. But you might be amazed to know that the symptoms I listed above are actually those associated with magnesium deficiency in children…not ADHD. It seems like doctors are quick to diagnose kids with ADHD when they experience symptoms that may simply stem from a variety of nutrient deficiencies. Isn't it ironic that a child with a magnesium deficiency may act a lot like a child who has been diagnosed with ADHD?

From The University of Maryland Medical Center – *Children with ADHD may be showing the effects of magnesium deficiency. In one preliminary study of 75 magnesium-deficient children with ADHD, those who received magnesium supplements showed an improvement in behavior compared to those who did not receive the supplements.*

My purpose in writing this chapter is not to convince you that all doctors and medicine is bad. As I said earlier, I do believe that there is a time and place for pharmaceutical drugs and I certainly encourage everyone to see their doctor for check-ups. I feel that our society has become lazy and it is so easy to blindly follow what we are told. I encourage everyone to do research and discuss options with your doctor and then make the decision you feel is best based on your research.

Modern medicine has failed us in many ways but health is a journey that is never too late to begin. The failures above are only a few of many and I believe that we can only achieve optimum health when we learn to provide our body with the nutrition it needs. When we get sick, we are not deficient in a pharmaceutical drug…we are out of balance and deficient in some nutrient most of the time. Pharmaceuticals only cover up symptoms. They don't heal us…only our body has the ability to repair and heal itself.

Summary

- Modern medicine and pharmaceutical drugs do have a place in our healthcare. The discovery of penicillin, certain vaccines, and surgeries have saved and extended millions of lives.
- Doctors often ignore the underlying causes of a disease.
- The medical establishment has a financial interest in suppressing the symptoms of disease rather than addressing the cause.
- Pharmaceutical drugs are responsible for at least 106,000 deaths per year.
- There is an effort, paid for by the medical establishment, to discredit safe, natural remedies.
- Americans are expected to blindly follow whatever we're told by the medical establishment.

Action Plan

- Do your own research and make an informed decision about your health. It is okay to question the advice of the medical establishment. Ultimately, you are in control of your health so do research and discuss what you learn with your doctor.
- There are many natural, safe nutritional supplements to address pain, cholesterol, and ADHD:
  - Pain Management: Curcumin, Ginger, Cannabis, CBD oil
  - Cholesterol (triglycerides): Berberine, Fish oil, ketogenic diet
  - ADHD: Magnesium, Low sugar diet, Physical activity

From Dr. Blair's Blog

It's NOT the gluten (it's the glyphosate)!

Over the past several years I've heard more and more people claiming an allergy to wheat gluten. I've wondered why, after consuming wheat for hundreds of years, many have developed this allergy over the past 10-15 years. What I found out is disturbing!

The practice of spraying glyphosate (RoundUp) on wheat crops started in the 1980's and became a regular practice in the 1990's. Farmers spray the crops to speed the drying process and improve crop yield. Glyphosate has been classified as a carcinogen and kills the friendly flora in the human gut leading to celiac disease, leaky gut, and weakened immunity.

Gerald Wiebe (Agriculture consultant) believes the use of glyphosate on wheat may be connected to the rise in celiac disease. "We've seen an explosion of gluten intolerance," he said. "What's really going on?" There are many reports of people with celiac and gluten intolerance having no issues eating wheat when traveling to countries like Italy where the use of glyphosate is banned! So is it a coincidence that celiac and gluten intolerance has become an issue during the time span that the spraying of RoundUp on wheat crops has become common, or are we being poisoned slowly by glyphosate? It's not the gluten...It's the glyphosate!

2

Unleash Your Inner Health

"Our Entire Lives Change in a Moment!"

— TONY ROBBINS

Now for the fun part of our journey. This chapter is about unlocking and unleashing the body's remarkable ability to heal. I will discuss the role that the mind plays in being healthy. I'll cover the reasons behind epidemic obesity and disease and provide an easy-to-follow program that will unleash your inner health. This book is 25 years in the making and if you'll give me a moment, you can change your life!

The human body desires balance. It is called homeostasis and our body craves it.

Homeostasis ho·me·o·sta·sis (hō'mē-ō-stā'sĭs) noun.
- The ability or tendency of an organism or a cell to maintain internal equilibrium by adjusting its physiological processes.
- The processes used to maintain such bodily equilibrium.

An easy to understand example of homeostasis is that the body maintains an internal temperature of 98.7 degrees despite the temperature around us. If the body temperature varies from that 98.7 the body is out of balance and usually fighting an invader such as a virus or bacteria.

Every year hundreds of new books hit the market about weight loss, diet, health, and fitness yet Americans continue to get fatter and sicker. The obesity rate has risen from 20% in 1980 to 65% today. Despite declaring "war" on cancer and heart disease they continue to be the number 1 killers. People put forth great effort and money to research "cures" but the statistics don't lie. This chapter is about reclaiming your health and changing who you are. As always, do your own research and make an informed decision about your health but it must start with your mind! Let's train your body to be healthy in an unhealthy world.

Have you ever wondered why the latest diet fads never work? There are several reasons for this but mainly because they do not address the two most important things...The underlying, root cause of the weight gain and the mental aspect of change. Later in this chapter I will address the root cause and give you an action plan to address it but first let's discuss the power of the mind.

A Healthy & Fit Body Begins Between the Ears

The first thing you must do in order to change your circumstance is re-define who you are. I recently spoke with a lady that had struggled for years with being overweight and she, like so many, told me that she had tried countless diets and exercise programs but that the weight always came back. Then she said something that told me who she really is. She said "I've always been fat so I guess I'll always be fat". If you think of yourself as a fat person then that's who you are but if you re-define yourself and change how you see yourself then you can have success.

It is not enough to set goals for yourself. We have been taught over the years by diet and health gurus to set goals and try to achieve them. Try? Instead of setting goals and hoping they are reached, raise your standards. Change is 90% mental and 10% effort, meaning if your brain is convinced it can be done then it will get done. Many years ago as a young powerlifter trying to bench press a lot of weight to win a trophy, I would tell myself over and over again "Get your mind right" before my big lift. I would mentally determine that I could lift the weight I was about to attempt and usually be able to do it…but it started in my mind. Later in life as I became a competitive runner, I would come up with things to say to myself before and during runs that would mentally prepare me for the grueling torture of running. I'll discuss my love/hate relationship with running later in the book.

If you want to lose weight, prevent or fight disease, lower blood pressure, reduce chronic pain, and have more energy then you have to mentally re-define yourself, raise your standards, and finally change your routine. If your daily routine is to get up, eat a crappy breakfast, go to a stressful job, come home to a stressful house and eat a crappy dinner, then watch TV or YouTube videos for hours before going to bed exhausted without having done any physical activity… you will be unhealthy. But if you change that routine because you've re-defined yourself as a fit, healthy person and raised your standards to accept nothing less than health and fitness, you will unleash your inner health! I know from experience that willpower doesn't work and cannot be relied on.

Willpower will always fail you but if you change your routine and re-define who you are you will succeed.

It is estimated that we have over 60,000 thoughts each day. 95% of those thoughts are the same thoughts we had yesterday, and the day before that, and the day before that. And most of the thoughts we have, whether positive or negative, elicit specific physical responses. Success begins and ends between your ears and there is a ton of research to prove it.

- One study looked at whether the relationship between exercise and health is moderated by one's mind. 84 female maids working in seven different hotels were measured on physiological health variables affected by exercise. Those in the informed condition were told that the work they do (cleaning hotel rooms) is good exercise and satisfies the Surgeon General's recommendations for an active lifestyle and examples of how their work was exercise were provided to them. Subjects in the control group were not given this information. Although actual behavior did not change, 4 weeks after the intervention, the informed group perceived themselves to be getting significantly more exercise than before. As a result, compared with the control group, they showed a decrease in weight, blood pressure, body fat, and body mass index. These women **thought** they were exercising and consequently lost weight, despite the fact that they were doing nothing out of the ordinary whatsoever. Crum et al. (2007)

- Another study tracked 105 obese people. 62 of them participated in three hours of cognitive therapy per week for ten weeks, while the others were in the control group. Cognitive therapy helps isolate negative thoughts, such as "I cannot lose weight" or "I will always be fat." 18 months after the therapy ended, those in the cognitive therapy group had lost an average of 23 pounds, while the control group gained an average of 5 pounds. Beck et al. (2005)

- One study wired test subjects up to weight machines that monitored levels of electrical activity in their biceps. Subjects were then asked to think in two different ways while exercising. One was not targeted while the other was specific to how the muscle was feeling and functioning during the movement. Researchers found that the subject's muscles worked more when they focused on what the muscles were doing. Results indicated that potentially greater strength would result from engaging in this practice of putting your "mind in your muscle." Marchant et al. (2005)

- Scientists in South Africa discovered something interesting about fatigue: It doesn't begin in the muscles. You know that burning feeling you get in your muscles toward the end of a hard workout? It comes from your mind. Biopsies of exhausted marathoners showed plenty of glycogen (the muscle's main fuel) and ATP (cellular energy source) despite the fact they were totally exhausted. Their conclusion: Fatigue sets in not when your muscles run out of gas, but when your brain tells them to conserve energy.

And here is one of my favorites:

- Australian psychologist Alan Richardson chose three groups of students at random. None of them had any experience with visualization. The first group practiced free throws every day for 20 days. The second group basically did nothing at all and the third group spent 20 minutes every day visualizing free throws with no practice at all.

  20 days later, the group that practiced daily improved 24%. The second group didn't improve at all. But the visualization only group improved 23% — statistically as much as the group that actually practiced! Richardson later noted that the most effective visualization occurs when the participant both feels and sees what they are doing in their mind prior to any physical engagement.

The studies above prove how powerful the mind is in health and healing. If you can raise your standards and change your routine you will achieve the health that your body craves. You must decide to be healthy before you will be healthy! Now that we know that health actually begins between our ears, let's look at some important dietary and supplement choices to unleash your inner health.

I've Tried Every Diet & Exercise Program

Almost every day I have someone tell me that they have tried every diet and exercise program and still cannot lose weight and keep it off.

Every year Americans spend millions of dollars on the latest fad diet craze and still our waistlines grow. You can visit your local book store and see entire sections with rows and rows of diet books and there are thousands of weight loss books available on Amazon. I'm frequently asked to lecture on diet and weight loss because the obesity rate is at epidemic level despite spending millions of dollars each year.

First let me say that I am not just an expert on nutrition but I am also someone that struggled with being overweight and dieting much of my life. I, like so many of you, tried every new diet program and supplement that I could and I hit the gym for a workout every chance I could. It wasn't until I discovered the principles I will share with you here that I finally lost the weight I needed to and have kept it off. At 50 years of age I am in the absolute best shape and health of my life so it's <u>never</u> too late to begin your journey to optimum health and fitness! I do not use the word "diet" when counseling a client because "diets" always fail.

I am not a proponent of the typical diet plan and I will not have you counting calories or eating things you don't want to eat. I will not lay out a plan here detailing what you should eat and at what time you should eat it. There are thousands of books that do that and it's just too hard to stick to those kinds of plans. Weight loss diets will always fail unless these 3 principles are followed:

1. **Re-define who you are and raise your standards!**
2. **Reduce "white" from your daily diet.**
3. **Reduce the stress hormone cortisol.**

I have already discussed the powerful role that our minds play in health and fitness and I will discuss stress in the next chapter. So let's talk about the harmful "white" stuff.

As I said, for many years I exercised and thought I was eating a healthy diet but still struggled with my weight. I finally realized that I must <u>decide</u> to be healthy and fit before I could <u>be</u> healthy and fit. I re-defined who I was and raised my standards. Doing this allowed me to change my daily routines and not rely on will power. Our entire lives change in a moment and for me that was my moment! Once I "got my mind right" the rest was easy (or at least easier).

The most harmful substances in our daily diets are "white". That includes sugar, bread, pasta, and potatoes. The typical American diet is loaded with whiteness and it is the leading cause of obesity and diabetes. We have been told (falsely) over the past 25 years or more that we need to avoid fat in order to lose weight and be healthy when it's sugar that's causing all the problems. As discussed earlier, our bodies need fat and cholesterol to simply survive, much less be healthy. But let's look at what happens when we eat too much "white".

In a perfect world it would be okay to load up on carbs because the body would shovel them into the muscles to be used as fuel to get us through a busy day of physical activity. But in today's world so many people are inactive that the carbs cause great damage instead of fueling us through the day. Now let me stop here for a minute and say that I do not promote a no-carb diet like Atkins. There obviously are benefits to some carbs like those in fruits and vegetables. I'm talking here about cutting down on "white" carbs and it is possible to do once you convince yourself that your new standard for yourself is to be slim, fit, and healthy!

When we eat white carbs our liver converts it to glycogen to be sent to muscles for fuel. When it gets to the muscle it is turned away because the muscle doesn't need it due to our inactive lifestyles. It's as if the sugar (glycogen) knocks on the muscle's door and asks to come in but the muscle says "there's no need for you here because we are not used enough". Once the muscle tells the sugar to go away it is sent back to the liver for reassignment. The sugar is told by the liver to "get back out there and find a home" so it searches for a place to stay. The search doesn't take long though. While the muscle cells have "no vacancy" signs lit up, the fat cells have their vacancy signs shining brightly! The fat cells are saying we want you if the muscles don't!

Eventually, even the fat cells have a hard time taking in the sugar and the liver converts the remaining sugar to fat in the form of triglycerides. If you have high triglycerides in your blood there is a good chance it's due to eating too many "white" carbs. The triglycerides then become dangerous when oxidized leading to heart disease. A simple way to explain oxidation is to cut an apple and let it sit out on the counter. It will turn brown as the oxygen begins to damage the delicate cells of the fruit. Oxygen does similar damage to our cells unless we have enough anti-oxidants in our diets to counteract that damage. It is oxidized (damaged) cholesterol and triglycerides that lead to heart disease.

Okay, back to sugar and white carbs. When I decided to greatly reduce (not eliminate) white carbs from my daily routine the fat began melting away. In the absence of carbohydrates the liver will convert fat into substances called ketones to be burned as fuel. The liver pulls fat from the cells and from the bloodstream to keep up with the production of ketones to fuel the brain as well as daily activity. This is the lifestyle I follow and recommend. A low-carb, ketogenic diet will burn fat and lower dangerous amounts of triglycerides and it is the only proven way to permanently lose weight and keep it off. If you add exercise to this scenario as I do, the body burns the fat even faster. Exercising on a typical high-carb diet doesn't usually work because you're just attempting to burn the carbs you eat and not the stored fat. I will discuss my fat-busting exercise routine later in the book.

As I said earlier, I will not give you a "diet program" to follow. There are thousands of those available and usually fail because they don't address the 3 principles above. Here is a typical daily routine for me:

- Eggs and sausage for breakfast with pomegranate juice: Eggs are one of the healthiest foods and this gives me protein and fat to fuel my morning with very few carbs. We will discuss the amazing healing properties of pomegranate next.
- A mid-morning whey protein shake or bar: This gives me more protein to fuel my day and not feel hungry

- A chicken or turkey sandwich for lunch: Yes, on a bun! This is my one indulgence of the day and 1 bun doesn't throw my routine out of balance.
- A mid-afternoon whey protein shake, bar, or boiled egg
- High-fat/protein dinner with steamed vegetables

I try to keep my daily carbs to around 50 grams to keep my fat-burning ketones working. The typical American diet contains well over 300 grams of carbs and that is the leading cause of obesity, diabetes, and heart disease. Notice that with the exception of a bun there were no white carbs. No white sugar, bread, pasta, rice, or potatoes. I do allow myself an occasional "cheat" meal but I try to follow my routine pretty well. It is easy to do since I re-defined who I am and want to be! My mind is in control of what I want to be and the direction I want to go.

Eat More Of These:

- **Eggs:** Excellent source of protein, brain-healthy fats, and vitamins.
- **Dark Chocolate:** Powerful heart-healthy antioxidant protection
- **Salmon:** Excellent source of protein and omega-3
- **Broccoli:** Source of cancer-fighting compounds called DIM & I3C.
- **Almonds:** Source of magnesium. Studies show almonds reduce risk of heart attack.
- **Green Tea:** Loaded with heart-healthy, cancer-fighting antioxidants.
- **Whey Protein:** Contains all essential amino acids. Aids tissue repair. Boosts glutathione (powerful antioxidant). Boosts immune function.

The body desires to be healthy and balanced and there are several ways to harness and unleash that desire. First, get your mind right.

Second, follow a low-carb, high fat, high protein lifestyle. Reduce the stress hormones which we will tackle in the next chapter, and incorporate some of nature's most powerful healing foods into your daily routine.

Health Benefits of: Pomegranate Juice

Research from around the globe confirms pomegranate is one of nature's most concentrated sources of antioxidants. Extraordinary findings indicate that compounds in pomegranate can do what scientists once thought to be virtually impossible— reverse the process of atherosclerosis.

These studies indicate pomegranate exhibits unprecedented cardiovascular protection by restoring endothelial health, lowering blood pressure, and protecting low-density lipoprotein (LDL) from damaging oxidation. Pomegranate also appears to fight several of the most common forms of cancer, slowing the progression of prostate cancer and suppressing the growth of colon, breast, and lung cancer cells. Pomegranate even appears to shield against unsightly signs of aging by supporting the health of the skin's underlying matrix. This is the closest nutrient I've studied to nature's fountain of youth elixir.

Pomegranate Enhances Nitric Oxide & Improves Endothelial Function

Endothelium Health: The cause and progression of vascular disease is intimately related to the health of the inner arterial wall. Blood vessels are composed of three layers. The outer layer is mostly connective tissue and provides structure to the layers beneath. The middle layer is smooth muscle; it contracts and dilates to control blood flow and maintain blood pressure. The inner lining consists of a thin layer of endothelial cells (the endothelium), which provides a smooth, protective surface. Endothelial cells prevent toxic, blood-borne substances from penetrating the smooth muscle of the blood vessel.

Many factors, including age, poor diet and those pesky free radicals, if left unchecked, will damage the delicate endothelial cells. This damage leads to endothelial dysfunction and ultimately allows lipids and toxins to penetrate the endothelial layer and enter the smooth muscle cells. This results in the initiation of an oxidative and inflammatory cascade that culminates in the development of plaque deposits. These plaques begin to calcify and, over time, become prone to rupture. If a plaque deposit ruptures, the result is oftentimes a deadly blood clot. As plaque builds up on the interior vessel walls they become partially or fully blocked, leading to sudden cardiac death.

Pomegranate protects cardiovascular health by enhancing nitric oxide production, which supports the functioning of the endothelial cells that line the arterial walls. Nitric oxide signals vascular smooth muscle to relax, thereby increasing blood flow through arteries and vessels. Nitric oxide reduces injury to the vessel walls, which also helps prevent the development of atherosclerosis.

An Italian study examined the role of pomegranate juice in nitric oxide activity in artery sections that had already developed atherosclerosis. The researchers selected mice with a genetic predisposition to developing atherosclerosis. They put the mice on a high-fat diet, let arterial disease develop for six months, and then added pomegranate juice to the experimental group's drinking water for 24 weeks. The placebo group was given plain drinking water.

Pomegranate juice not only increased the production of nitric oxide in both healthy and atherosclerotic blood vessels, but increased it the most in blood vessels with the most plaque buildup. In healthy parts of the blood vessels, pomegranate juice reduced vessel damage by nearly 26%, while in areas with much more plaque, pomegranate reduced vessel damage by approximately 20%.

Reversing Plaque Buildup

For years, scientists have believed that while antioxidants and other nutrients can slow additional atherosclerotic plaque buildup, they do little to reverse the process once plaque has already formed on the arterial walls. A remarkable study from Israel indicates pomegranate can actually reduce existing plaque formations in the arteries.

Nineteen patients from the Vascular Surgery Clinic in Haifa, Israel, were selected to participate in this three-year trial. All participants were non-smokers between the ages of 65 and 75, with severe carotid artery narrowing ranging from 70% to 90% blockage. In other words, their arteries were so obstructed by plaque buildup that only 10-30% of the original artery volume was available to permit blood flow. Ten of the nineteen patients consumed about 2 ounces of pomegranate juice daily, while the other nine received a placebo beverage.

Despite the patients' advanced atherosclerosis, consuming pomegranate juice produced significant reductions in the thickness of their carotid artery walls, which is correlated with decreased risk for heart attack and stroke. After only three months, the average thickness declined by 13%, and after 12 months, the thickness dropped 35% compared to baseline. During this same 12-month period, the average carotid artery thickness of the placebo group increased by 9%.

This study also measured various other parameters of cardiovascular health. One year of pomegranate consumption reduced systolic blood pressure by 21%. Systolic blood pressure refers to the maximum arterial pressure when the heart beats. Pomegranate intake appears to clear so many obstructions in the carotid arteries that the blood encounters less resistance, enabling the heart to pump at a reduced pressure. Less pressure through a wider "pipe" results in a lighter workload on the heart.

Total antioxidant content in the blood was increased by 130% after 12 months of pomegranate use, while oxidation of LDL cholesterol was reduced by 59%. Since LDL must be oxidized before it can adhere to the arterial wall, a reduction in oxidation and increasing levels of antioxidants in the blood can keep new plaque from building up.

The Israeli study also showed pomegranate consumption must be continued or the benefits are lost. Based on this research, I believe everyone should make pomegranate juice a part of their daily diet. It is the single best nutrient to keep the "pipes" clean and reduce vessel damage caused by poor diet, lack of exercise, toxins and exercise induced arterial damage.

Action Plan: The Israeli study used about 2 ounces daily of pure concentrated pomegranate juice. I believe the optimum dose is 4-8 ounces daily consumed on its own or as a delicious addition to a smoothie.

Jiaogulan Tea (Gynostemma)

During a country-wide census in 1972 it was discovered that a village in southeastern China had a population of people living routinely into their 100's. It was determined that their secret to longevity was jiaogulan (Gee-Ow-gu-lon), a climbing vine in the cucumber family that these people drank daily as a tea. The first written history of drinking jiaogulon was in 1406 and is known throughout China as Xiancao (immortality herb). Modern studies have shown jiaogulon to be a powerful anti-oxidant and immune-system stimulator. It has proven benefits as a heart tonic improving circulation and reducing blood pressure. It is consumed by villagers in the mountainous regions of southeast China and Taiwan to increase energy and endurance before work and to relax in the evening.

In the 1970s, while analyzing the sweet component of the jiaogulan plant, Dr. Masahiro Nagai discovered chemical compounds identical to some of those found in Panax ginseng, an unrelated plant. Later, Dr. Tsunematsu Takemoto discovered that jiaogulan contains four chemicals (saponins) identical to those in Panax ginseng as well as seventeen similar saponins. In total, 82 saponins were identified in jiaogulan, compared to only 28 found in Panax ginseng, making jiaogulan a more powerful superfood than ginseng.

Studies indicate jiaogulan stimulates the release of nitric oxide in the endothelium thereby lowering high blood pressure. In a double-blind study, gypenosides from jiaogulon administered to those with hypertension showed that 82% of the study participants reported lower blood pressure.

Other studies show jiaogulon increases heart-stroke volume, coronary blood flow, and cardiac output while reducing the heart rate, without affecting arterial pressure. In other words, this amazing plant has the ability to <u>make the heart stronger</u>, pump more blood with less pressure, and get more oxygen rich blood to all parts of the body faster. Here are the known benefits of jiaogulan:

1. **Powerful Antioxidant**
2. **Powerful Adaptogen (reducing stress hormones)**
3. **Enhances cardiovascular function (makes heart stronger)**
4. **Lowers High Blood Pressure**
5. **Prevents Heart Attack & Stroke**
6. **Strengthens Immunity**
7. **Supercharges Energy and Endurance**

This plant has been shown to increase the production of super oxide dismutase (SOD) by as much as 282%! SOD is the most powerful anti-oxidant known and contributes to fighting cancer and other disease. Jiaogulan is also the most powerful activator of the body's fat-burning, lifespan extending enzyme called AMPK.

Adenosine Monophosphate-Activated Protein Kinase (AMPK)

Every one of our trillion cells contain a master switch that basically controls that cell's health. The "switch" is responsible for the lifespan of the cell and is an enzyme called AMPK. All cellular functions and life are dependent on enzymes and AMPK may be the most important of them all. AMPK is like the guard at the door of each cell. Its main function is to regulate what goes into and out of each cell including fat and glucose. It also tells the cell when it's time to take out the garbage and clean house, keeping the cell young and healthy. Numerous studies show that activating cellular AMPK can extend the lifespan of each cell and therefore help prevent degenerative disease.

As we age our cells produce less AMPK leading to:

- Elevated blood sugar
- Chronic inflammation
- Increase in abdominal fat

- High triglycerides
- Weakened immunity

The research on activating AMPK is remarkable. A study published in 2013 in Cell Metabolism showed that AMPK activation can increase life span by up to 30%. It also improves glucose uptake into the cells and lowers blood sugar and triglycerides. AMPK also signals fat cells to release its fat stores to be used as energy resulting in weight loss.

There are a few ways to increase cellular AMPK. High intensity exercise like the kind I will discuss in a later chapter increases it as does calorie restriction. When you restrict calories the body increases AMPK as a tool for the body to function more effectively under stressful conditions. And finally there are some herbal supplements proven to increase AMPK activity. One of the most studied natural supplements for this is jiaogulan. The studies on jiagulan and AMPK are astounding.

One study from 2012 (Gauhar Hwang et al) showed:

- **8% reduction in body weight**
- **15% reduction in abdominal fat**
- **2 times more fat burning**
- **33% reduction in triglycerides**
- **20% lower glucose levels after meals**

Another study reported in 2014 (Park and Kim et al) was even more impressive. Over a 12 week period a group of obese people either took a jiaogulan supplement or placebo. At the end of the study those taking jiaogulan had lost an average of 3 square inches of total belly fat and an average of 1 inch in belly circumference. In other words, Jiaogulan is an effective fat burning aid through its mechanism of activating AMPK.

Action Plan: Jiaogulan is one of my favorite teas and I enjoy a cup or two every day. The studies above used a 450mg standardized extract of the leaf daily. I recommend a combination of both as the tea is tasty, rejuvenating, and refreshing.

Cannabis

The most powerful healing plant on the planet is also the most demonized. From the movies "Reefer Madness" to "Cheech and Chong" and many other "stoner flicks", marijuana has gotten a bad name. But let's take a look at the other side of marijuana, or cannabis. Cannabis has been used as a medicine and recreationally for several thousand years and has a remarkable history of safety and efficacy. Modern science has confirmed what I've known for many years…cannabis is a powerful healing plant! The historical use of cannabis goes all the way back to…The Bible!

The word for cannabis in the Bible is kanehbosm, also rendered in traditional Hebrew as kaneh or kannabus. The root kan in this construction means "reed" or "hemp", while bosm means "aromatic". This word appears five times in the Old Testament; in the books of Exodus, the Song of Songs, Isaiah, Jeremiah, and Ezekiel.

> *"Then The Lord said to Moses, "take the following fine spices: 500 shekels of liquid myrrh, half as much of fragrant cinnamon, 250 shekels of __kanehbosm__, 500 shekels of cassia – It will be the sacred anointing oil".*

> – EXODUS 30

Cannabis was an important part of the anointing oil and ceremonies of the Old Testament. Not only did God feel it should be part of anointing, He made cannabis a part of our design. In 1990 it was discovered that the human body has an endocannabinoid system located throughout. It has also been shown that the human brain has a large number of these cannabinoid receptors and they are there before birth in order to aid in brain development. Our bodies were designed to use cannabinoids for health, growth, and development from birth.

So what is a cannabinoid? They are a group of compounds that act on the cannabinoid receptors in the body and are unique to cannabis. The endocannabinoid system in the body is responsible for maintaining homeostasis, or balance. As I wrote earlier, our bodies have a desire for balance and health and cannabinoids are used for this purpose. In other words, **cannabinoids seek out problems in the body and fixes them.**

According to a 2013 study published in the British Journal of Clinical Pharmacology, cannabinoids have the following medicinal properties:

- **Anti-Inflammatory (reduce inflammation)**
- **Anti-Cancer**
- **Antioxidant**
- **Anticonvulsant (Suppresses seizure)**
- **Antidepressant**
- **Analgesic (pain relief)**

I encourage you to do your own research on this and not blindly follow the establishment telling you that cannabis is dangerous. Why is such a powerful healing plant still illegal in most areas of the United States? The answer of course is profit. The medical establishment including the FDA and government agencies refuses for the most part to acknowledge and approve cannabis despite its remarkable record of success in treating many diseases. But the doctors that refuse to acknowledge the healing power of cannabis are all too willing to prescribe a poisonous pharmaceutical drug.

Our government is two-faced on this issue. On one hand the government says that cannabis is a dangerous schedule 1 drug with NO medicinal value. On the other hand, the government holds US Patent #6630507 titled "Cannabinoids as antioxidants and neuroprotectants". It reads:

"Cannabinoids have been found to have antioxidant properties useful in the treatment of a wide variety of diseases, such as inflammatory and autoimmune diseases and to have application as neuroprotectants in the treatment of neurodegenerative disease".

So yes…the government knows that cannabis is medicine but is forced to demonize it and suppress it in favor of pharmaceutical sales. And we blindly follow…

Modern research proves that cannabis is a valuable tool in the treatment of a wide range of modern ailments. Marijuana is also a powerful appetite stimulant, specifically for patients suffering from HIV, the AIDS wasting syndrome, or dementia. Recent research suggests that cannabinoids and terpenes found in cannabis work together synergistically to help protect the body against some types of malignant tumors.

More than 60 U.S. and international health organizations including the American Public Health Association, Health Canada and the Federation of American Scientists support granting patients immediate legal access to medicinal marijuana under a physician's supervision. Others, including the American Cancer Society and the American Medical Association support clinical research trials so that physicians may better assess cannabis' medical potential.

A 1991 Harvard study found that 44% of oncologists had previously recommended marijuana to their patients and 50% said they would do so if marijuana was legal. A recent national survey performed by researchers at Providence Rhode Island Hospital found that nearly half of physicians surveyed supported legalizing medical marijuana.

Cannabis and its psychoactive cannabinoid THC, are considered incredibly safe for human consumption. The Drug Awareness Warning Network Annual Report, published by the Substance Abuse and Mental Health Services Administration (SAMHSA) contains a statistical compilation of all drug deaths which occur in the United States. According to this report, there has never been a death recorded from the use of cannabis! In fact, many studies show it is physically impossible for a human to die from a cannabis overdose.

The documented use of cannabis as a safe and effective therapeutic botanical dates to 2700 BC. In the 19th century, American journals of medicine published more than 100 articles on the therapeutic use of cannabis and cannabis was part of the American pharmacopoeia until 1942.

The cannabis plant has been around since the beginning of time. It is believed to have originated in Central Asia and people all around the globe consume cannabis because it makes them feel better.

We know that humans have cannabinoid receptors housed inside the body that are ready to bind with cannabinoids found in the cannabis plant to provide therapeutic benefits for a variety of ailments. In fact, cannabinoid receptors are present in humans before birth and cannabinoids are even found in a mother's breast milk. Our bodies are naturally tuned to interact with cannabinoids.

Cannabinoid receptor sites in the brain before birth suggests that the compounds could play a role in brain development. Cannabis has been linked to the creation of new neurons in the brain, or neurogenesis and is believed to have neuroprotective properties. Cannabinoids in marijuana actually help the brain grow through neurogenesis where new brain cells are constantly being created. A recent study from Italy showed that a cannabinoid called cannabichromene (CBC) can boost the growth of developing brain cells.

Another study published in The International Journal of Neuropharmacology stated that cannabidiol (CBD) is a key contributor of neurogenesis in the brain. Specifically, this birth of new neurons occurred in the Hippocampus, an area typically associated with conscious memory and navigation. By making these developing cells stronger, the chances for developing depression, Alzheimer's, and dementia are greatly reduced.

Daily doses of tetrahydrocannabinol (THC) seemed to improve short-term memory in the subjects, compared to those that were left untreated. Additionally, those receiving THC showed signs of greater learning ability.

"Daily doses of tetrahydrocannabinol (THC) seemed to improve short-term memory in the subjects, compared to those that were left untreated."

-Dr. Irit Akirav

Cannabis can also protect the brain from chronic daily stress. Everybody suffers from some sort of stress in their day-to-day lives. Stress can take its toll on your emotional state, but it can also change the way your brain works over time. Stress is also one of the most common causes of anxiety and depression, a growing problem we face as a nation. According to research from Israel, cannabis may protect your brain from the effects of constant stress. Researchers found that "cannabinoid receptor activation could represent a novel approach to the treatment of cognitive deficits that accompany a variety of stress-related neuropsychiatric disorders". What this means is that the cannabinoids found in marijuana protect against the disorders associated with daily stress.

Many studies have proven that cannabinoids have anti-cancer properties. Spanish researchers from Complutense University found that tetrahydrocannabinol (THC) was actually able to kill brain cancer cells. After administering THC to mice with human tumors, researchers found that THC actually caused the tumor to shrink.

Dr. Peter McCormick from UEA's School of Pharmacy in Dubai, who co-lead the study with researchers from Complutense said "Our findings help explain one of the well-known effects of THC on tumor growth. Although it has been proven that cannabis oil can reduce the size of tumors, cancer patients should always consult their doctor"

Research shows promise for THC in cancer treatment, but many are skeptical of using THC-based products because of its psychotropic effects (high). As a result many practitioners have redirected their focus toward cannabidiol (CBD) and cannabigerol (CBG). A recent British study, however suggests that cannabinoids may be most effective against cancer when acting synergistically with one-another. In other words, the whole plant is more effective than part of the plant.

Action Plan: This is a tough one because it involves politics. The evidence is clear that cannabis is a powerful healing plant with remarkable safety and efficacy. The medical establishment and government tell us that this is a dangerous drug yet no one has ever died from a cannabis overdose! On the other hand, "legal" drugs like alcohol, tobacco, and pharmaceuticals are responsible for hundreds of thousands of deaths each year. If you believe that cannabis should be legal, especially medicinally, then get involved and contact your state representatives. Educate your friends and family to start breaking away the stigma and demonization. It is outrageous that a weed that grows naturally and has powerful healing properties is responsible for filling the jails of this country. Even more outrageous is that it is kept from the sick people that it might heal!

Beet Root

I must admit before I even write one word that I have never eaten a beet! I had an experience at my cousin's house when I was around 10 years old that made me hate beets before I ever tasted one. I walked into my cousin's house and smelled the worst smelling stench I had ever smelled. When I asked what that smell was I was taken to the kitchen where I saw beets being cooked on the stove and I swore that I would never eat that vile food! And I never have. Having confessed that, I have consumed beet juice and beet root powder for its health benefits. The beet root is a rock star in the health and nutrition world!

The history of beets dates back to ancient times, and the earliest signs of their cultivation were around 3,000 years ago in the Mediterranean region. From there, beets were transported to Babylon, and by the 9th century AD, they had made their way into Chinese culture and cuisine. They have long been associated with improved sexuality and have been used as an aphrodisiac for thousands of years. Beets have such a wide range of health benefits because of their nutritional content, including vitamins, minerals, and organic compounds like carotenoids, lutein/zeaxanthin, glycine, betaine, dietary fiber, vitamin C, magnesium, iron, copper and phosphorus. They are also a source of beneficial flavonoids called anthocyanins.

Beets are rich in nitrates, which the body converts to nitric oxide, a compound that relaxes and dilates blood vessels, improving blood flow and circulation. Better circulation means lower blood pressure. A study from 2012 (Lundberg, J.O.; Carlström, M.; Larsen, F.J.; Weitzberg, E.) found that those who drank just one glass of beet juice daily lowered their systolic blood pressure by an average of 4 to 5 points. Another study published in Hypertension in 2008 found that those who drank beet juice had a 10 mm Hg drop in blood pressure and less blood clotting three hours later, compared to those who drank water.

Beets don't just have a positive impact on your blood pressure. They are also rich in a plant alkaloid called betaine, as well as the B-vitamin folate, which together deliver a one-two punch for lowering blood levels of homocysteine, which in high levels increases your risk for artery damage and heart disease.

Beet juice can also help increase endurance. In one study, cyclists who drank beet juice could pedal hard 15% longer in a time trial to exhaustion. It takes about three to five beets (a cup of beet juice) to get the performance boost, says study author Andy Jones, PhD, dean of research in the College of Life and Environmental Sciences, University of Exeter. "Peak nitrate levels occur two to three hours after you eat or drink them," he says. So time your intake accordingly if you want to crush your 5K PR.

Nitric oxide relaxes and dilates your blood vessels, which in turn increases blood flow to the brain, which could improve brain function. That's particularly important as we age, as research finds that our capacity to generate nitric oxide diminishes as we get older, along with our brain's energy metabolism and neuron activity. So give your brain a boost with beets. In one small 2010 study, 14 older men and women (average age of 74) who ate a high-nitrate diet, including beet juice, for two days enjoyed more blood flow to the frontal lobe of their brains, a region known to be involved with skills like focus, organization, and attention to detail.

The liver does the heavy work of cleaning your blood and detoxifying the body. You can lighten its load with a daily serving of beets.

Research shows that betaine, an amino acid found in beets (as well as spinach and quinoa) can help prevent and reduce the accumulation of fat in the liver. A study showed that those given beet juice have higher levels of detoxifying enzymes in their bloodstream. Research on people with diabetes shows that betaine improves liver function, slightly decreases cholesterol, and reduces liver size.

Beets are also rich in betalains, a class of potent antioxidants and anti-inflammatories that battle free radicals and inflammation related chronic diseases like heart disease, obesity, and possibly cancer.

Action Plan: Drink 100% beet root juice every day. I mix 2 spoons of beet root powder in water and drink it.

Curcumin

For several thousand years Indian cultures have incorporated turmeric into their daily diet and reaped the health benefits that come with it. Many modern studies have proven what the people of India have known all along...turmeric can help prevent heart disease, cancer, high blood pressure, inflammation and pain, Alzheimer's and dementia, diabetes, and much more.

Research is also showing that turmeric is not absorbed and utilized very well and that it takes a lot of turmeric to get the health benefits. Curcumin however is the golden pigment in the turmeric and has proven to be better absorbed. Curcumin is also where most of the beneficial compounds are located. Curcumin has proven antioxidant, anti-inflammatory, and anti-cancer properties. According to research, curcumin not only prevents oxidative damage to artery walls, it can also heal damage already done. And as we will discuss, curcumin can tell a cancer cell that it's time to die. Curcumin is also one of the most powerful anti-inflammatory nutrients known...reducing not only the inflammation in joints causing pain but also throughout our circulatory system and brain.

Heart disease is still the number one killer in the United States but according to an Indian study curcumin can raise HDL (good) cholesterol as much as 29%. It is the HDL form of cholesterol that grabs onto excess fats and cholesterols in the bloodstream and escorts them back to the liver for disposal. That's why HDL is called "the good cholesterol". Curcumin also reduces the inflammation which is a leading cause of heart disease. Researchers at Peter Munk Cardiac Center in Toronto report that curcumin can dramatically reduce the instances of heart failure. Curcumin is a powerful antioxidant that can prevent the oxidative damage to the arteries and actually heal damage already done, making it a potent heart healthy food.

Cancer is the number two killer in the United States despite our medical establishment waging "war" on it and spending trillions of dollars to find the cure! According to research from prestigious institutions like Sloan-Kettering Cancer Center, curcumin can play a big role in preventing and even fighting cancer. According to the journal Anticancer Research, curcumin can suppress tumor growth and spread. It can do this by blocking a cellular enzyme that helps cancer invade cells, and by cutting off blood supply to tumors.

The number one reason reported that people visit their doctor these days is for pain relief. Thanks to our diets and sedentary lifestyles, inflammation has taken over our bodies. This inflammation is a leading contributor to heart disease, diabetes, cancer, dementia, and pain! As we discussed earlier, too many people turn to NSAIDS or prescription opioids to manage their pain and these can be very dangerous. Typical pain relieving medications work by blocking the inflammatory enzyme called Cox-2. The problem is that these medications also block the beneficial enzyme called Cox-1. Cox-1 is an enzyme needed for healthy digestion and circulatory health so blocking it can be dangerous. Curcumin has been shown to suppress the harmful Cox-2 enzyme without affecting Cox-1, meaning it can reduce the pain-causing inflammation without affecting digestion and circulation.

Type 2 diabetes is a modern disease created 100% by lifestyle. In fact, type 2 diabetes has increased by over 75% in the past 25 years… about the same rate as obesity. Heart disease and diabetes go hand-in-hand and heart disease is actually the number one killer of diabetics. Diabetes can increase blood pressure and increase the risk of dying from heart disease or stroke. According to a Columbia University study, those given a daily dose of curcumin were less likely to develop diabetes, and an Indian study showed that curcumin can help lower blood sugar, increase insulin sensitivity, and repair damage done by hyperglycemia.

Alzheimer's and dementia are devastating diseases that are unfortunately on the rise as we continue to eat inflammatory diets and reduce cholesterol. The brain simply cannot function without cholesterol and our typical diets are loaded with inflammation-causing omega-6 fats. Curcumin has been shown to reduce the inflammation in the brain as well as the beta-amyloid plaques that build up. These are plaques that build up around the neurons and prevent proper signaling. Curcumin has the ability to cross the blood-brain barrier and heal the conditions leading to dementia and Alzheimer's.

Action Plan: Curcumin is a remarkable spice that should be incorporated into everyone's daily routine for its antioxidant and anti-inflammatory benefits. Cook with turmeric for some benefit (and 'cause it tastes delicious), but take a curcumin supplement daily for the health benefits.

Kombucha Tea

In case you haven't figured out by now, I enjoy drinking some funny sounding drinks! My three favorite health drinks are Kava, Jiaogulan, and kombucha. I drink a fair amount of Chinese green tea as well but there are hundreds of books already discussing the health benefits of green tea.

The first recorded consumption of kombucha was in ancient China around 221 BC. Over the centuries since then it has become a popular health promoting drink throughout the orient as well as in Russia and Germany. Kombucha's popularity in the U.S. has been growing in the past several decades as people learn of its amazing health properties.

So what exactly is kombucha and why is it so healthy? The origin of the name kombucha is up for debate but the best explanation I have found is a Japanese translation of "kombu" meaning brown algae and "cha" meaning tea. So is it a brown algae tea? It certainly looks like it is but modern science has revealed what it truly is and has confirmed many of the historic health benefits.

Many physicians, nutritionists, and herbalists know the health benefits of eating fermented foods such as yogurt, kefir, tempeh, and sauerkraut. These foods are beneficial because they contain natural enzymes and friendly bacteria that are alive. Our bodies were designed to utilize "live" foods for nutrition and the typical American diet contains little to no "live" foods.

Kombucha is a fermented, "live" drink made from tea and sugar. I know I told you earlier to avoid sugar but as you'll see in a minute, the fermentation process eliminates most of the sugar in kombucha. So, kombucha is made by combining tea (black, oolong, or green) with cane sugar and a symbiotic colony of bacteria & yeast (SCOBY). The SCOBY actually digests the sugar in the mixture turning it into a fermented, probiotic drink. The process takes about 8-10 days and the SCOBY can be re-used many times for several years.

Kombucha tea is loaded with antioxidants called polyphenols. These polyphenols can fight free radical oxidation and is a weapon against modern diseases like heart disease and cancer. It is a powerful liver detoxifier and has a history of helping people with digestive issues. Even former President Ronald Reagan drank kombucha as part of his diet when he was fighting colon cancer in 1985.

Kombucha's health benefits come from its antioxidant content as well as a high amount of probiotics and acids. Probiotics (meaning pro-life) are necessary for proper digestion as well as a strong immune system. The acids found naturally in this drink aid in digestion and utilization of minerals and in the detoxification and health of the liver. These acids also possess antibacterial properties.

Action Plan: There are numerous historical health claims and folk tales about the healing benefits of kombucha. I simply drink it daily as a healthy, "live" food that provides friendly bacteria, antioxidants, and enzymes to my diet. It is a low sugar, carbonated, rejuvenating and refreshing drink.

Cordyceps Mushroom

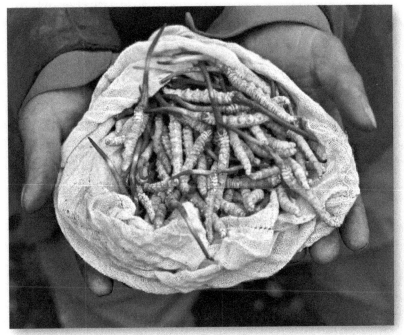

Wild harvested cordyceps mushrooms

Cordyceps is a mushroom that grows in the high Himalayan altitudes of Tibet and has been used in Chinese Medicine for several thousand years. It is called caterpillar fungus because in the wild it grows from dead caterpillar carcasses and was once reserved only for Chinese Emperors. Traditionally, cordyceps has been consumed for its many benefits to the heart and lungs, for its energy-boosting effects, and for anti-aging purposes. Modern science is verifying all of these uses, and more. In human cardiovascular studies, use of cordyceps lowered serum triglycerides and cholesterol overall, and increased beneficial HDL (good cholesterol) levels. Cordyceps enhances nutritional blood supply to the organs and extremities and defends the heart against exercise stress.

Cordyceps enhances respiration and the body's use of oxygen, and helps to improve cases of chronic asthma and bronchitis. It also possesses antioxidants which retard cellular destruction, and has anti-inflammatory properties. Cordyceps also helps to protect the liver and kidneys from environmental damage.

Cordyceps can help to turn back the aging clock as well as super-charge endurance and energy!

In a number of competitive events, winning Chinese athletes have attributed their elite performance in part to regular use of cordyceps. Their competitive success led to the study of cordyceps for energy, endurance and stamina. Analysis of cordyceps reveals natural substances which boost immunity, increase stamina, and improve recovery from fatigue. It has been proven to speed the transfer of oxygen from the bloodstream to the cell which for endurance athletes means optimal Vo2 max performance (oxygen uptake). Heisman Trophy Award winner and 11-year NFL star running back Ricky Williams told me that as he got older he often used cordyceps for the additional energy boost during a game.

In elderly patients, cordyceps improved a number of quality of life parameters, including general physical condition, mental health, appetite, vitality, sexual drive and cardiac function. In effect, cordyceps can help to turn back the aging clock as well as super-charge endurance and energy!

Action Plan: Cordyceps is one of my favorite herbs. The research is clear that cordyceps can enhance endurance and performance and I attribute it to helping me personally reach new levels of fitness. I prefer taking it in capsule form (although if you're ever in the high mountains of Tibet you may search for it growing in dead caterpillars on the side of the mountains).

Summary

- A healthy and fit body begins between the ears.
- Change is 90% mental.
- To accomplish any goal you must re-define yourself and raise your standards!
- Sugar & simple carbohydrates (bread, pasta, potatoes, rice) are the causes of weight gain, obesity, heart disease, diabetes, and inflammation.
- "Diets" will always fail. Change your lifestyle and mental attitude to lose weight and achieve the life you desire.

Action Plan:

- Set aside 30 minutes per day for motivation and discovery. Use this time to watch an inspiring video on YouTube or read a motivational book. This time will help you focus on re-defining who you are and who you want to be.
- Reduce sugar and simple carb consumption! It is all about moderation. It is okay to "cheat" occasionally and indulge in a sweet treat or have some potatoes, but as you continually strive to raise your standards and re-define yourself it will become easier to avoid them.
- Find a way to incorporate most (if not all) of the following into your daily diet:
  - Pomegranate Juice
  - Jiaogulan Tea
  - Cannabis (where legal of course!) CBD oil
  - Curcumin
  - Kombucha Tea
  - Cordyceps Mushrooms
- Eat a high fat / moderate protein / low carb diet (see Blair Diet next)

The Blair 21 Day Weight Loss Diet

I do not like the word "diet" but it is a word ingrained in our daily vocabulary. Every year, Americans spend millions of dollars on the latest fad diets and programs while getting fatter and fatter. The Blair 21 Day Diet is **not** a typical, calorie restrictive diet that frustrates and fails millions of people yearly. Diets fail because they do not address the underlying **cause** of weight gain, and because they are impossible to maintain. The typical diet plan is simply too restrictive to be realistic on a long term basis. It's not realistic to believe that you can maintain extreme calorie restriction long term. When you restrict calories to 800 to 1000 as many popular diets do, you may lose weight but do you really want to eat like a small bird the rest of your life?

It has been shown that it takes at least <u>21 days to form a habit</u> so I encourage you to give this at least 21 days. The Blair Diet does not restrict total calories…just the ones that count. Weight loss is a lifestyle change where the power of positive thinking is just as important (if not more important) than what we eat. Willpower is not enough to insure success. It is important to change the way you think about your daily routine. Instead of saying "I <u>should</u> lose weight" or "I <u>should</u> eat fewer sweets", make it a <u>must</u>! You are more likely to accomplish your goals if you <u>must</u> do it. The mind is a powerful tool in permanent weight loss and health. Redefine who you are and change your daily routine and Unleash Your Inner Health!

The key to effective fat loss is to reduce certain carbohydrates, including white sugar, white potatoes, white bread, white pasta, and white rice. The key word here is…white. I believe that permanent weight loss is possible without starving yourself (with calorie restriction) by reducing the white things in our diets. I follow a ketogenic diet that forces the body to burn fat in the absence of sugar. By reducing white carbohydrates, the liver produces ketones made from fat to burn as fuel. Where does the liver obtain the fat needed to make these ketones? To make ketones the liver pulls fat from several places, including the bloodstream (triglycerides) and fat stores throughout the body. A ketogenic lifestyle is the most effective diet plan for fat loss and optimum health. With the Blair 21 Day Diet you will not be hungry…making success more attainable. Here is a guide to an effective Blair keto diet:

Breakfast

Pick one: **Pick one:**

- Eggs (2-3)
- Sausage   **AND**
- Bacon
- Beef
- Chicken
- Turkey

- Natural almond butter
- Natural sunflower butter
- High fat / low sugar yogurt
- Sausage
- Bacon
- Low sugar protein bar

Drink unsweetened green, oolong, or jiaogulan tea, coffee, or water

Morning Snack (Pick One)

- Low-sugar protein bar
- ½ cup of almonds or walnuts
- ½ cup of sunflower seeds

Lunch

Pick One: **Pick One:**

- Chicken
- Beef
- Turkey   **AND**
- Eggs
- Salmon
- Tuna

- Steamed Broccoli
- Carrots
- Green beans
- Avocado
- Kale / Spinach salad*
- Whole grain bun or bread if you want a sandwich

Drink unsweetened tea, kombucha, or water

Afternoon Snack (Pick One)

- Low-sugar protein bar
- ½ cup of almonds or walnuts
- ½ cup of sunflower seeds
- Low-sugar whey protein shake
- Apple

Dinner

Pick One: **Pick Two:**

- **Chicken**
- **Beef**   **AND**
- **Turkey**
- **Ham**
- **Salmon**
- **Tuna**

- **Steamed Broccoli / Cauliflower / Green beans / Spinach**
- **Kidney/Pinto/Black beans**
- **Avocado**
- **Kale / Arugula / Spinach salad***
- **Carrots**
- **Green Beans**
- **Peas**

Drink unsweetened tea / green, oolong, or jiaogulan tea, or water

Occasional Evening Snack (Pick One)

- Whey Protein Shake
- Buttered Popcorn (1/2 cup)
- 1/2 ounce Dark Chocolate (about 2 bites)

*Check labels and be sure to use a low-sugar dressing. Olive oil & vinegar are good choices.

Supplements for Weight Loss

- **Adrena-Live**: An adaptogenic herbal formula to reduce the stress hormone cortisol. High cortisol levels increase appetite and belly fat.
- **Berberine**: Balances blood sugar and increases AMPK activity. AMPK is an enzyme that regulates the amount of fat a cell can hold.
- **Jiaogulan**: Increases AMPK activity.
- **Green Tea**: Contains EGCG which increases metabolism.
- **MCT oil**: A saturated fat that increases ketones to be used as fuel. Ketones will help you maintain energy while on a keto-genic low-carb diet.

Guide to Eating Out

- **Choose Low-Carb selections if possible**
- **Avoid French Fries at fast-food restaurants**
- **Push the dessert menu away**
- **Watch portion sizes (restaurants often super-size portions)**
  - **Get a box and take some home**
- **Choose fruit as a side dish**

Things to AVOID

- **High Fructose Corn Syrup (more harmful than sugar)**
- **Diet sodas containing aspartame:** Aspartame suppresses serotonin which <u>increases</u> appetite. It can also cause seizures and decomposes into formaldehyde.
- **Trans Fats** (hydrogenated & partially hydrogenated oils)
- **Soy protein:** Soy protein can suppress thyroid function.
- **Canola Oil:** An omega 6 oil that is highly inflammatory.
- **Negative thoughts & Self Doubt!**

The Blair 21 Day Weight Loss Diet is an easy-to-follow lifestyle change that does not overly restrict calories and zap your energy. The key to success for any healthy lifestyle is between the ears…meaning a strong mental attitude. When you redefine who you are through meditation, visualization, and motivation you will have greater success. Remember that you cannot rely on willpower…it usually fails you. Set goals that you must accomplish and visit those goals every day. Incorporate a "cheat" meal occasionally and do not be discouraged if you fall to occasional temptation…just get back on schedule quickly. Weight loss and optimum health is a journey, and every journey begins with the first step. Enjoy and embrace the journey!

From Dr. Blair's Blog

Vitality of a Horse (ashwagandha)

Ashwagandha is one of the most powerful herbs in Ayurveda (traditional Indian medicine) and has been used for 2500 years for a wide variety of conditions. It is well known for its restorative benefits. In Sanskrit (Hindu) Ashwagandha means "vitality of a horse," indicating that the herb promotes the vigor and strength of a stallion, and has traditionally been prescribed to help people regain energy, reduce stress, and strengthen the immune system. Ashwagandha is frequently referred to as "Indian ginseng" because of its rejuvenating properties although botanically, ginseng and Ashwagandha are unrelated.

Ashwagandha is considered a rasayan herb in Ayurveda meaning it's a promoter of life. Medical researchers have been studying Ashwagandha for many years with great interest and have completed more than 200 studies on the healing benefits of this herb. Some proven examples of the healing effects of Ashwagandha are:

- Restores youthful energy and endurance
- Strengthens and protects adrenal function
- Strengthens the immune system
- Helps combat the effects of stress (reduces cortisol)
- Improves learning & memory
- Reduces anxiety and depression
- Helps reduce brain-cell degeneration
- Stabilizes blood sugar
- Anti-inflammatory
- Enhances sexual potency for both men and women

If you are one of the millions of people that suffer from daily fatigue, carbohydrate craving, fat accumulation around the belly, insomnia, sexual dysfunction, and/or a weakened immune system then this Ayurvedic rock-star herb with a strange name might be the rejuvenative herb you need.

3

They Saw A Warrior (The Stress Connection)

Those living on the islands in the south Pacific are called "the happiest people on Earth". Of course with a warm, sunny climate and beautiful beaches it makes perfect sense that they would be happy! But they also have a 3000 year old secret to their happiness…kava.

For 3000 years the villagers living on the south Pacific islands of Vanuatu, Fiji, Samoa, and Hawaii have consumed the root of a local plant in ceremonies, meetings, special occasions, and just to relax. Kava was discovered and first written about by Captain James Cook while exploring the south Pacific in the late 1700's. He wrote about "an intoxicating pepper" that today is referred to as "the root of happiness". The islanders drink kava nightly to relax. They drink kava at village meetings, ceremonies, to settle arguments (it is said the "it is impossible to hate with kava in you), and to welcome people traveling through.

On one occasion a large, tattooed, black man walked into a village on the island of Samoa. The villagers welcomed him and the Chief decided to have a kava ceremony to welcome their guest. He sent some men into the forest to pick fresh kava roots. They then ground the roots, mixed it with water and strained the juice into a large bowl. At the ceremony, everyone sat around this large bowl of what looked like muddy water and took turns drinking it from a hollowed coconut shell. The Samoan villagers that day did not see a famous American football player, or a Heisman Trophy winner. They did not see a "quitter", or a "pot head" as he has been called by some in the media. They did not see a man that has had the weight of an entire city on his shoulders after being drafted number 5 overall in the NFL draft when the team that drafted him had given up their entire draft to get him. They did not see a man with social anxiety disorder that has a brilliant mind and wants to be known for more than scoring touchdowns. That day, in the Samoan village, **they saw a warrior!**

In 1998 I began watching the University of Texas football games because my favorite college coach was in his first year there. Mack Brown had left my UNC Tarheels for Austin, Texas to coach the Longhorns. I knew nothing of the Longhorns but as a fan of Coach Brown I knew they had a coach that would care deeply about the football program, the school, the fans, and most importantly the players.

The first game I watched on TV that year I noticed a running back for Texas that reminded me of another Longhorn running back that I had grown up watching named Earl Campbell. I had been a huge fan of Earl Campbell and thought that this running back had his size and power, but was much faster! He was going to be fun to watch. His name was Ricky Williams and the first game of the season he blew up for 215 yards and 6 touchdowns! The next game he ran for 160 yards and 3 more TD's! 6 more touchdowns against Rice then 5 against Iowa State on his way to 2,129 rushing yards, 28 touchdowns, the all-time college rushing record, and the Heisman Trophy! I had become a Longhorn fan and a Ricky Williams fan that year.

At the NFL draft the New Orleans Saints and their coach Mike Ditka traded away their entire draft to move up to the number 5 pick to draft Ricky. The expectations and weight of the entire city now rested on the shoulders of this shy, soft spoken kid from southern California. The first two seasons in New Orleans was disappointing as the weight of expectations and 350 pound defensive linemen came crashing down leading to injuries and ultimately manifesting in social anxiety. I watched as sports reporters interviewed Ricky with his helmet on and no one trying to understand the immense pressure this young man had on him to perform…to win…to be a hero! He ran for 884 yards his first year with the Saints but only scored 2 touchdowns in 12 games. The next year was slightly better as he rushed for 1000 but again was injured. Still feeling the pressure and wearing his helmet during interviews Ricky began to "self-medicate" with marijuana.

In 2001 Ricky played an entire season for the first time as a pro and had a good year statistically, but the Saints were going nowhere and he was traded to my Miami Dolphins. 2002 was an all-pro year for Ricky as he led the league in rushing yards with 1853 and 16 touchdowns! The Texas Tornado, Heisman Trophy winner, all-time greatest collegiate rusher had finally arrived as the NFL star he was destined to be! And the pressure continued to mount. The toll physically was immense as he carried the ball an NFL most 383 times that year, then 392 times the following year. But the toll mentally was still adding up as well as now Ricky had the pressure of continuing to have to live up to the growing expectations. And the "self-medicating" continued.

I will never forget the day I heard the news! It was like when people remember where they were the day Kennedy was assassinated, or the day Elvis died. I turned on Sports Center one morning as I ate my breakfast just in time to hear, "Ricky Williams retires"! How could that be? He's the stud running back for my favorite team! He's a superstar now! He's got everything and he's walking away from it all!

We all know the story now. Ricky "retired" to avoid another suspension for failed drug tests. He used his retirement to travel and "find" himself. He lived in a tent in Australia where he read books about life, religion, and philosophy. He lived in a rental house in Grass Valley, California and studied the ancient healing of Ayurveda. And yes, it was Ricky Williams that wandered into the village in Samoa.

Ricky came back to play five more years in the NFL with the Dolphins, then retired with the Baltimore Ravens in 2012. As a Dolphins fan I felt betrayed by Ricky when he suddenly retired before that season. But I became an even bigger fan of Ricky Williams because of it! He has been able to control his social anxiety disorder with yoga,

Ayurveda, medical cannabis, kava, and finding consciousness. We will discuss all of those and more in this book.

I am honored to have gotten to know my favorite football player! Ricky Williams is much more than a remarkable athlete and I believe he will ultimately be remembered more for what lies ahead. Ricky Williams is a warrior…a philosopher…a healer…a teacher…and most importantly to me, my friend.

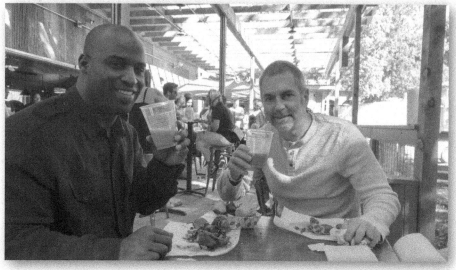

Ricky Williams and I drinking Kava at a Nakamal (kava bar)

The Stress Connection

Most people never feel the stress of being a pro football player, but we all deal with some form of stress in our daily lives. I have been studying the effects of daily stress since my Doctoral research beginning in 1999. Imagine for a moment that you are a gazelle in the African plain. You are drinking water from a small pond when you notice a lion creeping up on you. Your adrenal glands kick into high gear flooding your circulatory system with adrenaline and cortisol and you take off running.

After a brief chase the lion gives up and you are out of danger! You immediately go back to grazing and drinking as if nothing happened. That is how the adrenal glands are supposed to work. Excrete enough of the stress hormones into the blood to get you through a dangerous situation.

The difference between us and that gazelle is that as soon as the stressful situation has passed, the gazelle goes about its business as usual. It does not, as we do, dwell on it…text about it…tell its friends about it…or post it on Facebook or Tweet about it! We have a hard time "letting it go" and that puts more strain on our adrenal glands as we continue to live that stressful situation.

Laugh It Off!

"Laughter is the only medicine without side effects."

— SHANNON L. ALDER

Tina, a 38 year old mother of 2, gets up at the crack of dawn to get the kids ready for school. After dressing and feeding them she must get herself ready for work and get them to school on time. All morning, Tina is worrying about a project deadline looming at the end of the week that her boss is hounding her about. Her youngest child hasn't slept well in two nights due to a bad head cold and her oldest child is dealing with drama at school. As she rushes out the door with barely enough time to get to school on time, her office calls and tells her they will be short-staffed today and she will need to fill in at the receptionist desk along with her normal duties. Knowing time is of the essence, Tina takes a short-cut to school hoping to miss the normal morning traffic delays only to discover traffic on this route is at a standstill due to a fender bender!

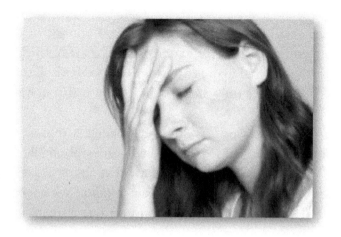

How many people reading this can identify with Tina? Men and women unfortunately deal with stress every day and that stress is slowly killing us. Stress, whether from work, school, children, traffic, or sickness, is the root cause of many illnesses and diseases. In the above example, Tina is a client I counseled after she came to me for weight loss advice. She told me she had tried several popular diets with little success and she had joined her local gym to exercise but she could only go sporadically. She simply didn't have the energy to go to the gym and she was frustrated by one failed diet after another. Tina suffered from the most prevalent condition of our time... exhaustion! More specifically adrenal exhaustion caused by stress.

Stress & Adrenal Glands

The adrenals are small kidney shaped glands that sit atop each kidney and play a huge role in our health. These tiny glands are responsible for controlling other glands such as the thyroid and pancreas as well as regulation hormones like testosterone, estrogen and progesterone. They are also the "stress" glands, responsible for getting us through stressful situations. Under stress, the adrenals release stress hormones into the blood stream to prepare the body for battle. These hormones are adrenaline and cortisol.

The adrenal glands are designed to release these stress hormones during acute times of need. In other words, when in fight or flight mode being robbed by a burglar or chased by a lion. They are not designed to handle the everyday stress of modern society and therefore are constantly being over worked.

Everyday stress causes the adrenals to release cortisol into the bloodstream and this constant infusion of the stress hormone is very detrimental to health. As cortisol attempts to "protect" the body from stress, it does several things that are ultimately harmful. Cortisol raises blood pressure causing the heart to pump harder and it signals fat cells to retain fat while causing carbohydrate cravings. In other words, cortisol causes weight gain and increases appetite. The old saying "desserts is stressed spelled backwards" makes perfect sense now!

The overworking of the adrenal glands set off a domino effect in the body. The adrenals are the master endocrine gland meaning they control the proper functioning of other glands. Overworked adrenals effects the proper functioning of other endocrine glands including the pancreas and thyroid and also affects the balance of the sex hormones estrogen, progesterone and testosterone. Stress induced overworked adrenal glands are the number one root cause of daily fatigue, weight gain, insomnia, mental and sexual dysfunction, and contributes to diabetes, heart disease, menopause and much more.

Action Plan

"Now I'm fighting cancer, everybody knows that. People ask me all the time about how you go through your life and how your day, and nothing is changed for me. As Dick said, I'm a very emotional and passionate man. I can't help it. That's being the son of Rocco and Angelina Valvano. It comes with the territory. We hug, we kiss, we love. When people say to me how do you get through life or each day, it's the same thing. To me, there are three things we all should do every day. We should do this every day of our lives. Number one is laugh. You should laugh every day.

> *Number two is think. You should spend some time in thought.*
> *Number three is, you should have your emotions moved to tears,*
> *could be happiness or joy. But think about it. If you laugh, you*
> *think, and you cry, that's a full day. That's a heck of a day. You*
> *do that seven days a week, you're going to have something special"*

— JIMMY VALVANO (LEGENDARY NC STATE COACH)

Laugh, think and cry! As coach Valvano said in his famous speech only weeks before he passed away, everyone needs to do those three things every day. Let's begin with the health benefits of laughter...

1. **Laugh**: Laughter, along with an active sense of humor, may help protect you against a heart attack, according to a study by cardiologists at the University of Maryland Medical Center in Baltimore. The study, which is the first to indicate laughter may help prevent heart disease, found people with heart disease were 40 percent less likely to laugh in a variety of situations compared to people of the same age without heart disease.

   It is known stress is associated with impairment of the endothelium, the protective barrier lining our blood vessels. This can cause a series of inflammatory reactions leading to fat and cholesterol build-up in the coronary arteries and ultimately to a heart attack. Laughing can greatly reduce the damaging effects of cortisol.

   In the study, researchers compared the humor responses of 300 people. Half of the participants had either suffered a heart attack or undergone coronary artery bypass surgery. The other 150 did not have heart disease. One questionnaire had a series of multiple-choice answers to find out how much or how little people laughed in certain situations, and the second one used true or false answers to measure anger and hostility. The most significant study finding was people with heart disease responded less humorously to everyday life situations.

They generally laughed less, even in positive situations, and they displayed more anger and hostility.

Daily laughter is also good internal exercise. It exercises the diaphragm, lungs and heart while releasing endorphins to improve mood. A good sense of humor is necessary for a strong relationship as well and my wife and I try to incorporate some laughter every day.

The evidence is clear that laughing can reduce stress and heart disease while increasing immunity and improving relationships. **Action Plan:** Laugh! Watch a comedy or read a funny book every day. Just laugh!

2. **Drink Kava:** Every herbalist has a favorite herb and mine is kava. Kava is a plant that grows in the south pacific and has been consumed both socially and as a medicine for several thousand years. Once reserved only for tribal chiefs, kava is now widely consumed around the world for stress and anxiety relief.

All kava comes from the south pacific islands of Vanuatu, Fiji and Hawaii. The root of the kava plant is ground, mixed with water and downed quickly. Why quickly? It tastes like muddy pepper water but many mix it with juice to make it taste better. Capsules are available but are not as effective.

So, why am I asking you to drink something that tastes bad? Because it is effective! There are numerous studies proving kava works well to reduce stress and anxiety but I'm going to focus on personal experience. I have been drinking kava almost nightly for many years and can say it is very effective.

The first thing noticed is an analgesic effect in the mouth, meaning it slightly numbs the tongue. This makes it a good remedy for tooth aches as well. The numbness is short-lived and harmless...I actually enjoy it. The second thing noticed is an almost instant feeling of calm. I can actually feel the stress of the day leave my body and I feel relaxed.

Two studies from Duke University prove kava's effectiveness and safety. One study determined kava is as effective for relieving anxiety as the benzodiazepine class of drugs (Valium, Xanax). The other study found no liver toxicity resulting from the use of kava.

Kava has proven to be a superior remedy for stress and anxiety, and an unrivaled relaxant. We can learn valuable lessons from the native people of the Pacific islands, who regularly enjoy the relaxing effects of kava, and use the occasion of drinking kava to put a leisurely end to the labors of the day and reflect on life. In our hectic, overworked, fast-paced world, reduced stress and greater relaxation can make us healthier and life more enjoyable. With or without the warm breezes and swaying palms of the Pacific islands, kava is one of nature's great plant treasures, a true elixir of relaxation.

Action Plan: Find a good source of south pacific kava and buy the instant powder. It mixes easiest with water. Mix one or two teaspoons of instant kava powder with 4- 6 ounces of water and drink it quickly. Mix with fruit juice to mask the taste if needed. I drink one or two cups every evening. If in Vanuatu, seek out a kava bar, or "nakamal". There are also a few nakamals spread throughout the United States.

3. **Take Ashwagandha**: No plant medicine is more prized in India than ashwagandha. It has been used as food and medicine for nearly 3000 years and has been studied extensively. Ashwagandha is used in India to treat daily fatigue, stress, mental exhaustion, sexual debility and insomnia. I recommend using it to boost endurance and energy but included it in this chapter due to its remarkable ability to help balance stress hormones by protecting the adrenal glands.

Ashwagandha is a plant that grows abundantly throughout India and it is the root of the plant that is consumed. I have included it in my stress relief supplements for over 12 years because it is the best supplement to take for adrenal protection, cortisol reduction, and exhaustion.

Action Plan: Ashwagandha root comes in capsules and tablets. I recommend 1000mg – 2000mg daily with a meal.

4. **Run Forest Run** (at least move): In the movie Forest Gump, Tom Hank's character loved to run! He ran everywhere, sometimes for days. What does Forest Gump have in common with marathon runners and joggers that run at least a mile a day? Less stress! Not less physical stress...we've already discussed the physical toll running can have on the body (and how to avoid it) but instead less emotional and hormonal stress. Simply putting one foot in front of the other on a regular basis relieves stress and anxiety and if you run long enough you'll experience the release of "feel good" endorphins, called the "runner's High".

Running is a fundamental part of leading a healthy and fit life. Even if you're in good health and fit, running needs to be a part of your lifestyle. The body just needs it. If you're overweight, there aren't many better ways to burn fat than by beating the pavement with a brisk walk or run. Running can help you shed as many as 100 calories per mile and aids in lowering your blood pressure by making sure the arteries stay smooth and elastic. In fact, running can cause your arteries to expand and contract as much as three times more than the arteries of someone who spends all his time sitting on the couch. Running also slows down the hands of time as regular runners are less likely to have bone and muscle loss. This is because as we age, bones can either grow stronger if they're worked out, or weaker, if you're a couch potato. The sedentary lifestyle can lead to osteoporosis. The active runner will remain strong and flexible.

Those are just a few of the physical benefits of running. As you probably figured, there are some psychological benefits for runners as well. Stress in both its forms, acute and long-term, have some pretty nasty effects on your body. Acute stress comes on fast and typically doesn't last very long. It can be triggered by anything, from an auto accident to bumping into an old flame you weren't prepared to see. Most of your body systems are negatively affected by acute stress. Your brain, lungs, heart, immune system and digestive system all ramp up to deal with whatever trigger got you so worked up, whether it's a real danger or just perceived. Long-term, or chronic, stress is even worse. Over time, your heart will have to work harder, and your immune system will weaken and cortisol will send fat straight to your waistline. Arthritis, heart disease, diabetes and aging all can be triggered by chronic stress.

If you lead a hectic and stressful life, running can help. Psychologically, running gives you a set amount of time to be alone with your thoughts. Use this to your advantage. You can use that time to get your brain around an issue at the office or the problem with your significant other. In studies, regular runners generally say they live a happier, more stress-free life than couch potatoes. Aside from simply being happier because you're in better shape and feeling good, endorphins play a big role in these results. You might know endorphins as the "feel-good" hormones of the body. It's an opioid chemical that the body uses to help relieve pain. They also help slow the aging process, relieve stress and anxiety, and enhance the immune system. Running can release a flood of these endorphins into the bloodstream so the next time you feel stressed, hit the road and run for 20 or 30 minutes. It is one of the best known stress-relievers available!

Action Plan: Head outside and run at least 15 minutes a day. For optimum stress relief benefits I recommend a minimum of 30 minutes at least three days per week. I recommend outside if possible to enjoy the benefits of sunshine and fresh air but if you must a treadmill works too.

Stress can have a very damaging effect on the body. The action plan I laid out can greatly reduce the damage of everyday stress and contribute to better health and happiness. In addition to these recommendations, consider incorporating additional nutrients into your daily stress relief routine including rhodiola, sea salt, and magnesium to protect against adrenal exhaustion and balance stress hormones.

Summary

- Ricky Williams brought social anxiety disorder to an entirely new audience when he was expected to carry the city of New Orleans on his shoulders.
- Most people do not experience the same stress as a professional athlete but we all deal with some form of stress every day.
- Daily stress is the leading cause of weight gain, fatigue, insomnia, weakened immune system, hormone imbalance, inflammation, and heart disease.

Action Plan

- Laugh every day! Find a show that makes you laugh out loud and watch it every day. Find a book or cartoon that makes you laugh and read it. Tell jokes with your spouse or children and act silly. Laughter is a key to stress reduction and a healthier life.
- Drink Kava. Kava is known in the South Pacific as the *Root of Happiness* and is proven to reduce stress and anxiety. It has a calming effect on the entire body.
- Take Ashwagandha and other adaptogenic herbs. These herbs have been proven to lower the stress hormone cortisol and protect the adrenal glands from daily over use.
- Exercise! Run or walk. Begin by taking a 10 minute walk every day until you build up to more. Re-define yourself as someone that is motivated to get up and move. Exercise will release "feel good" endorphins and make your heart healthier

From Dr. Blair's Blog

The Immortality Herb

Jiaogulan (Gynostemma pentaphyllum) is a low-lying vine from the Cucurbiticeae (cucumber) family of plants. Jiaogulan is indigenous to Southern China but is now cultivated widely throughout Asia, most notably in Thailand.

Traditional Chinese Medicine recommends Jiaogulan as a general health tonic and in southern China it is called Xian Cao (the Immortality Herb) due to its association with longevity and robust health.

Jiaogulan has been shown to increase the production of super oxide dismutase (SOD) which is the most powerful antioxidant in the human body. This may contribute to the long lifespans and vibrant health of those that consume it.

Researchers in Korea have determined that jiaogulan is a potent activator of the AMPK enzyme in humans. AMPK plays a crucial role in the regulation of human metabolism. In one Korean study, obese men were given jiaogulan extract for 14 weeks. The placebo group experienced no significant change. However the jiaogulan group lost an average of **4 pounds,** saw reduction in their waistlines, improved body mass index and lower cholesterol levels.

Jiaogulan should be part of a healthy diet and lifestyle for optimal health.

4

A Little Bit 'O Sunshine

(The Most Important "Vitamin")

"I cannot endure to waste anything so precious as sunshine by staying in the house"

- Nathaniel Hawthorne

The sun: It not only provides the earth with light and heat, it is necessary for life! Without the sun our bodies cannot produce what I think is the single most important vitamin, vitamin D. It is involved in every cell and research is showing many Americans are deficient in vitamin D and that deficiency is leading to heart disease, cancer, weakened immunity, weak bones and much more. So let's begin with a quick lesson on Vitamin D.

Vitamin D 101:

Vitamin D is important for good overall health and strong and healthy bones. It's also an important factor in making sure your muscles, heart, lungs and brain work at optimum levels and keeping the immune system strong to fight infection. Your body can make its own vitamin D from sunlight but we can also get vitamin D from supplements and a very small amount comes from a few foods we eat.

The vitamin D that comes from sunlight and the vitamin D from supplements has to be changed by the body a number of times before it can be used. Once it's ready, the body uses it to manage the amount of calcium in your blood and bones and to help cells all over your body to communicate with each other properly.

What does vitamin D do?

The link between vitamin D and strong, healthy bones was made many years ago when doctors realized that sunlight, which allows you to produce vitamin D, or taking cod liver oil, which contains vitamin D, helped to prevent a bone condition called rickets in children. Today, vitamin D is seen as a vital part of good health and it's important not just for the health of your bones. Recent research is now showing that vitamin D may be important in preventing and treating a number of serious, long term health problems. Vitamin D isn't like most vitamins. Your body can make its own vitamin D when you expose your skin to sunlight. But your body can't make other vitamins. You need to get other vitamins from the foods you eat. For example, you need to get vitamin C from fruits and vegetables. Also vitamin D is unique compared to other vitamins in that it is actually a hormone called "activated vitamin D" or "calcitriol."

Vitamin D is very important for strong bones. Calcium, magnesium and phosphorus are essential for developing the structure and strength of your bones, and you need vitamin D to absorb these minerals. Even if you eat foods that contain a lot of calcium and magnesium, without enough vitamin D, you can't absorb them into your body. Vitamin D is important for overall health, and researchers now are discovering that vitamin D may be important for many other reasons besides bone health. Vitamin D is necessary for:

- **Healthy Immune system**
- **Muscle function**

- Healthy heart and circulation
- Healthy lungs
- Brain development

Vitamin D deficiency has also been linked to other diseases such as cancer, asthma, type-II diabetes, high blood pressure, depression, Alzheimer's, and autoimmune diseases like multiple sclerosis and Crohn's. When the skin is exposed to the sun, vitamin D is produced and it is sent to the liver. The liver changes it to a chemical called 25(OH)D. When a doctor talks about vitamin D levels, he means the amount of 25(OH)D in your blood. This chemical is then converted into "activated D" to be utilized by every cell.

How to get Vitamin D

The two main ways to get vitamin D are by exposing your skin to sunlight and by taking vitamin D supplements. You cannot get the right amount of vitamin D your body needs from food.

The best way to obtain vitamin D is by exposing your skin to sunlight (ultraviolet B rays). This can happen very quickly particularly in the summer. You don't need to tan or burn your skin to get vitamin D. You only need to expose your skin for about 15-30 minutes. How much vitamin D is produced from sunlight depends on the time of day, where you live in the world and the color of your skin. The more skin you expose the more vitamin D is produced.

The skin can make large amounts of vitamin D when it is exposed. The body is designed to get the vitamin D it needs by producing it when your skin is exposed to sunlight. The part of the sun's rays that is important is ultraviolet B (UVB). This is the most natural way to get vitamin D. You don't need to tan or to burn your skin in order to get the vitamin D you need. Exposing your skin for a short time will make all the vitamin D your body can produce in one day. In fact, your body can produce 10,000 to 25,000 IU of vitamin D in just a little under the time it takes for your skin to turn pink. You make the most vitamin D when you expose a large area of your skin, such as your back, rather than a small area such as your face or arms.

You can also obtain vitamin D by taking supplements. This is a good way to get vitamin D if you can't get enough sunlight, or if you're worried about exposing your skin. Vitamin D3 is the best kind of supplement to take. It comes in a number of different forms, such as tablets and capsules, but it doesn't matter what form you take, or what time of the day you take it.

What's Cholesterol got to do with it?

Cholesterol is the most misunderstood substance in the body. For many years it has been vilified and made to be the primary cause of heart disease. There are many books, studies, and opinions on this subject and I will let you do your own research and come to a conclusion. Having said that, cholesterol is way too important to be such a villain. In fact, it is so important we simply cannot live without it! Every cell in the human body is made by cholesterol and every hormone is formed by it. How can something so critical to life be so bad?

Cholesterol is crucial to making vitamin D as well. In the skin UVB rays combine with cholesterol in order to form vitamin D. In other words, the two things we have been told over the past 25 years to be the most scared of, sunlight and cholesterol, actually make vitamin D. No wonder so many people are deficient in this absolutely vital vitamin.

Why Vitamin D?

- **Heart Disease:** Heart disease is a major problem for both men and women in the United States. Every year, approximately 715,000 Americans suffer a heart attack. About 1 out of every 4 deaths is a result of heart disease, which is the leading cause of death for men and women in the US.

Research has shown that vitamin D deficiency can actually increase your risk of heart disease. A recent Norwegian study found that people with the lowest vitamin D levels had a 32% greater risk of dying from cardiovascular disease than those with the highest vitamin D levels.

Each year, heart disease increases in prevalence in the United States. According to the American Heart Association, roughly 83 million American adults have at least some type of heart disease. Approximately 78 million have hypertension (high blood pressure), 15 million have coronary heart disease and 5 million have congestive heart failure.

Two types of heart disease that can be reduced by sufficient vitamin D are atherosclerosis and endothelial dysfunction. Atherosclerosis is characterized by the build-up of plaques in the arteries. These plaques often form when things like fat, cholesterol, and calcium accumulate in the arteries. These plaques make it more difficult for blood to flow throughout the body and therefore increase the risk for heart attack and stroke. Laboratory studies using human blood cells showed the activated form of vitamin D suppressed oxidation of cholesterol and diminished plaque formation.

Vitamin D supplementation has been shown to improve endothelial function. Endothelial function is critical to the smooth and easy flow of blood through the vessels and a dysfunctional endothelium can be a contributing factor for conditions such as coronary artery disease, hypertension, and diabetes. Vitamin D plays a vital role in keeping the heart strong and the blood flowing smoothly thus reducing the risk of heart disease.

- **Breast Cancer:** Studies have shown there is a link between vitamin D and breast cancer. Women who have breast cancer tend to have low levels of vitamin D in their body. Women with higher vitamin D levels are less likely to develop breast cancer. Women with higher vitamin D levels who already have breast cancer tend to have smaller tumors and are less likely to die from breast cancer.

Some studies have been done which have found women with low levels of vitamin D are more likely to develop breast cancer. A recent review of many studies found post-menopausal women with low levels of vitamin D had a higher risk of getting breast cancer compared to post-menopausal women with high levels of vitamin D.

Other studies have found what is called a dose-response relationship, where for each increase in vitamin D levels in the body; there is a decrease in breast cancer risk.

A Canadian study looked at a group of women with early stage breast cancer. The researchers looked at their vitamin D levels and followed them over 12 years to see how their cancers progressed. They found that:

o Women with low vitamin D levels were almost twice as likely to have their cancer spread to another part of the body than women with high vitamin D levels.

o Women with low vitamin D levels were more likely to have died during the study than women with high vitamin D levels.

o Women with low vitamin D levels had worse tumors than women with high vitamin D levels.

Vitamin D appears to play a vital role in reducing the risk of developing breast cancer and dying from it.

- **Colorectal Cancer:** Colorectal cancer is the third most common cancer in the United States and there appears to be a correlation between vitamin D levels and colorectal cancer rates. Places where people are exposed to the lowest amount of sunlight have higher rates of colon cancer than people in sunny places. Since sun exposure helps make vitamin D, researchers think that the higher rates of colon cancer may be due to low vitamin D levels.

A recent review of many studies found that high vitamin D levels in the body are linked to a lower risk of developing colon cancer. Another review found people with the highest levels of vitamin D were half as likely to develop colorectal cancer compared to people with the lowest levels of vitamin D. Other studies have found a dose-response relationship, where for each increase in vitamin D levels in the body, there is a decreased chance of getting colorectal cancer.

Vitamin D may play a part in preventing colorectal cancer and as vitamin D deficiency continues to rise so do the rates of cancer.

- **Prostate Cancer:** Prostate cancer is the second most common cancer in men and there appears to be a correlation between vitamin D levels and prostate cancer rates. A large study that followed men for 13 years found that those with the lowest levels of vitamin D had the highest risk of getting prostate cancer. Men with dark skin are more likely to develop prostate cancer, which may be because they need more sun exposure to make enough vitamin D, which is especially difficult in African American men.

  Another study followed American males for 18 years and found that the men with the lowest vitamin D levels had the most aggressive forms of prostate cancer. Researchers think that vitamin D might help to slow the progression of prostate cancer.

  An American study from 2012 looked at men with prostate cancer and followed them for 5 years. They found out how many men had died during that time and how many of their cancers spread to other body parts. The research showed men with the lowest levels of vitamin D had almost double the chance of dying from prostate cancer or having it spread to other body parts compared to men with the highest levels of vitamin D.

Prostate cancer is very treatable if diagnosed early. I include vitamin D in my arsenal to help prevent this dreaded disease.

- **Influenza**: Influenza, more commonly known as the flu, is a respiratory infection caused by a virus infecting the nose, throat, and lungs. Influenza is most common during winter and can cause fever, chills, sore throat, cough, body aches, fatigue and death. Vitamin D is an important part of the immune system. Some studies have shown that there is a link between vitamin D levels and the risk of getting influenza. People with low vitamin D levels may have a higher chance of developing influenza. Influenza epidemics occur in the winter when vitamin D levels are dramatically lower. Since influenza is seasonal, it is thought that vitamin D might be a factor that can affect your chances of getting the flu.

Some studies have shown taking vitamin D supplements can reduce your chances of getting influenza.

An experiment done with Japanese schoolchildren looked at the effects of vitamin D supplements on their chances of getting influenza. The researchers gave children either 1,200 IU vitamin D per day for 3 months during the winter, or a placebo. They found that more children in the placebo group got influenza A than children in the vitamin D group and there was a preventive effect of 1,200 IU vitamin D per day on children getting influenza A. The researchers concluded that taking 1,200 IU of vitamin D in children can help to protect against seasonal influenza.

Immune cells have vitamin D receptors and as discussed earlier, each cell needs to be turned on to work efficiently and vitamin D is the key that turns them on. There are many studies and many more conditions and diseases that vitamin D deficiency is linked to that an entire book could be devoted solely to the sunshine vitamin. Not really a vitamin, more of a hormone, vitamin D appears to play a role in heart health, immune health, cancer prevention and athletic performance.

- **Exercising:** For several decades it has been thought people performed better athletically in summer due to UVB exposure and now we know why. Many studies have confirmed that vitamin D is necessary for optimum athletic performance and endurance. One mechanism by which this happens is by increasing testosterone. Another is by making muscles work more efficiently. In one study, four Russian sprinters were doused with artificial, ultraviolet light. Another group wasn't. Both trained identically for the 100-meter dash. The control group lowered their sprint times by 1.7 percent while the UVB runners, in comparison, improved by an impressive 7.4 percent.

  Researchers at Louisiana State University conducted a study to determine if there was a relationship between vitamin D status and measures of body composition and physical fitness among students attending the university. Thirty-nine students with an average age of 23 years were recruited for the study. The researchers measured their vitamin D levels. To determine body composition and physical fitness, the researchers measured factors including body mass index (BMI), resting metabolic rate, maximal oxygen uptake (VO2max), and muscular strength. VO2max is a measure of the maximum rate of oxygen consumed during exercise and is an indicator of physical fitness. The researchers determined those with the highest vitamin D levels were the fittest, with the lowest body fat and highest Vo2max, while those with lower vitamin D levels were less fit.

  Low D levels might also contribute to sports injuries, in part because Vitamin D is so important for bone and muscle health.

In a Creighton University study of female naval recruits, stress fractures were reduced significantly after the women started taking supplements of Vitamin D.

A number of recent studies also have shown that, among athletes who train outside year-round, maximal oxygen intake tends to be highest in late summer. The athletes, in other words, are more fit in August, when ultraviolet radiation from the sun is near its strongest. They often experience an abrupt drop in maximal oxygen intake, beginning as early as September, even though they continue to train just as hard. This decline coincides with the autumnal weakening of the angle of sunlight. Less ultraviolet radiation reaches the earth and, apparently, sports performance suffers.

Every cell in the human body has vitamin D receptors, including muscle and heart cells, and vitamin D is the key that turns on each cell. In other words, the cell cannot function at peak levels unless vitamin D has turned it on. Just like a super powerful, clean, well-conditioned car engine cannot run with the key to turn it on, the body cannot run without the key.

Action Plan: For optimal health I recommend between 1000 IU and 5000 IU per day. I personally take 5000 IU per day. African American men and women may need a higher dose because they are generally more deficient than Caucasians.

Summary

- Vitamin D is more than a vitamin…it's a hormone
- There is a vitamin D deficiency epidemic in the United States because we have been told for 30 years to avoid the 2 things responsible for D production in our bodies…cholesterol and sunlight.
- Vitamin D is necessary for proper immune function and reduces the risk of heart disease and cancer.
- The African American population is at most risk of deficiency.

Action Plan

- Get 20 – 30 minutes of sun exposure every day.* The sun not only is responsible for the production of vitamin D, it makes you feel good too.
- Don't take cholesterol lowering drugs.* They are dangerous and they reduce the ability of the body to produce vitamin D.
- Take a vitamin D3 supplement. The Vitamin D Council recommends everyone take at least 5,000 IU daily. African American population may need more.

*Discuss with your doctor the benefits of sunlight and cholesterol and make an informed decision together.

From Dr. Blair's Blog

South Pacific Islanders Don't Suffer from Anxiety!

As an herbalist I've studied herbs in cultures from around the world and my favorite is kava. Kava (piper methysticum) is a small shrub native to the islands in the South Pacific. The root and stems are made into a non-alcoholic, psychoactive beverage that has been used socially and ceremonially for 3000 years in Vanuatu, Hawaii, Fiji, and Tonga. Kava is traditionally prepared by placing the ground root into a porous sack, submerging in water, and squeezing the juice into a large wooden bowl. Coconut half-shell cups are dipped and filled — punch bowl style. After drinking a cup or two a feeling of heightened attention combined with relaxation begins to come on. Unlike alcohol your thoughts remain clear.

Kava is a remarkable stress and anxiety reliever. It contains compounds known as kavalactones that operate on non-opiate pathways to offer a natural and non-narcotic action against anxiety. Some clinical research even suggests that they're as good or even better than pharmaceutical drugs like benzodiazepines.

According to Duke University Medical Center, kava is beneficial for anxiety and doesn't produce dependency or negatively affect heart rate, blood pressure, or sexual function. In a 75-participant, 6-week, double blind trial conducted by the University of Melbourne Department of Psychiatry, kava was found to reduce anxiety and was well tolerated.

If you start researching kava, warnings about liver damage are the first thing you'll see. This is a subject with much contention. The research indicates there is no evidence to support these claims. Both Ohio State University and the South Dakota State University College of Pharmacy conducted studies and found that kava is non-toxic to the liver and may even protect the liver.

So take the edge off the day with a shell (or capsule) of kava and enjoy the peaceful relaxation of the islands!

Tear this page out and post on refrigerator

Do These Things <u>Every Day for 21 Days</u>!

- Spend 20-30 minutes in motivational videos or books to raise your standards and define your success
- Research nutritional & herbal remedies to make informed decisions
- Laugh & Cry…or laugh until you cry
- Reduce sugar & white carbohydrate consumption
- Enjoy a "cheat" meal occasionally. Forgive yourself & refocus when you fail. Healthy living is a journey.
- Drink pomegranate juice, jiaogulan tea, & kombucha
- Take adaptogenic herbs such as ashwagandha for stress
- Take 5,000 IU Vitamin D3 for immune health
- Exercise! Get out and move. Walk 10-20 minutes or more. Build yourself up to a run if you can. Take a yoga class or do yoga at home.

Recommendations for Common Ailments

- Aches & Pains:
  Curcumin, Ginger, MSM, CBD oil
- Anxiety:
  Kava, Cannabis, CBD oil, L-Theanine
- Cold & Flu:
  Olive Leaf Extract, Neem Leaf, Oregano Oil, Boneset herb
- Bacterial Infection:
  Colloidal Silver, Berberine
- Constipation:
  Magnesium Oxide, vitamin C
- Candida:
  Berberine, Oregano, Probiotic
- Diabetes Type 2:
  Berberine, Neem Leaf
- Erectile Dysfunction:
  L-Arginine, Maca Root, Shilajit
- GERD (reflux):
  Digestive Enzymes, Betain HCL, DGL Licorice, apple cider vinegar
- Gout:
  Black Cherry Juice, Celery Seed
- Insomnia:
  Kava, Valerian Root, L-Theanine, Melatonin
- Irritable Bowel (IBS):
  Peppermint Oil
- Migraine Headaches:
  CBD oil, Magnesium
- Memory & Focus:
  Bacopa, Gotu Kola, Magnesium
- Menopause:
  Black Cohosh, Ashwagandha

- Restless Leg: Magnesium Malate
- Premenstrual Syndrome (PMS):Chaste Tree (Vitex), Ashwagandha
- Stress: Ashwagandha, Kava, Vitamin C
- Urinary Tract Infection (UTI): Cranberry Juice, D-Mannose

5

Why I Run (and why you should too)

"I always loved running…it was something
you could do by yourself, and under your
own power. You could go in any direction,
fast or slow as you wanted, fighting the wind
if you felt like it, seeking out new sights just
on the strength of your feet and the courage
of your lungs".

-Jesse Owens

"Daddy, where are you going?" my daughter Ashley asked me one cold, wet, Saturday evening as I was lacing up my running shoes. "Running," I said. "Why?" she asked.

It was a good question, and one I couldn't easily answer. I didn't really want to go. I could go later….or the next day. Or just not run at all. "Because it's fun," I said, rather unconvincingly. The truth is, just before you run is the worst possible moment to try to explain to someone, or even to yourself, why you run. It just doesn't make sense. Running is hard. It requires effort. And after all the pain you usually end up right back where you started, having run in a big, pointless circle.

People sometimes say to me they can run if they're chasing a ball or to escape from a vicious dog, but to just run, nothing else, just one foot in front of the other? Many find it just too boring and unnecessary. There is no logical reason to run. Of course, some people run to lose weight, or to get fit and reduce the risk of heart disease and diabetes, and these are great reasons. Running is relatively easy to do, it's cheap, and you can do it when you want without having to book a court or join a team. All these factors certainly contribute to the fact that running is one of the most popular sports in the world.

Many runners, including me, become obsessed with times. The need to break the 20-minute barrier for the 5K, for example, or run under 4 hours in a marathon, can become the reason we run. There is something reassuring about striving towards such fixed goals, measuring your progress in numbers that are not open to interpretation, but stand there as unambiguous achievements. And as soon as they are achieved, another target is thrown out almost instantly. The times themselves are not the reason we run mile after mile, up hills in the wind and rain. The times are merely the carrots we dangle in front of ourselves.

"Why do we do this to ourselves?" Why do we put ourselves through so much pain just to obtain a personal best or win a trophy? Deep down, we all know the answer... Running brings us joy! Watch small children when they are at play and they can't stop running. Back and forth, up and down. I remember as a child, I'd often break into a run when walking along the street, for no apparent reason. We were born to run according to a theory devised by Harvard scientists. They theorize that humans evolved doing long-distant hunting; chasing animals down until they dropped dead. It's why we have achilles tendons, arched feet and big gluteus maximus (butt) muscles. While even the fastest sprinter would be left behind in a race against most four-legged mammals, over long distances we are the Olympic champions of the animal kingdom. If they could keep them in sight for long enough, our ancestors could catch even the swiftest runners such as antelope just by running after them.

As children we just run. Sometimes we run to get home quickly when we're late for dinner. Sometimes for sport and sometimes...just to run! As adults, we seem to have lost that innate need and desire to run so we formalize it. We become runners! We buy new $150 running shoes and running clothes. We dangle our carrots (goals & targets), we download iPhone apps, and we sign up for races (so there's no backing out). And once everything is set up, finally we can run. Racing along out on the trails, or through the busy streets of a city! Splashing through puddles and letting the rain drench us and the wind chafe us, runners begin to sense a faint recollection of that childish joy! As we run, the layers of responsibility we have accumulated in our lives during that day or week; the father, mother, lawyer, teacher all melt away, falling to the ground with each drop of salty sweat, leaving us with a feeling of satisfaction, accomplishment and peace. In Japan, monks run marathons in an attempt to reach enlightenment. Many athletes try Iron Man or ultra-marathons to push their body to the breaking point and beyond. Some runners run for fitness or for a cool 5K t-shirt. What all of these runners feel after crossing the finish line is the same… It's the runner's high which of course may only be chemicals flooding the brain, but after a long run everything seems right in the world. Everything is at peace.

So we run because we were born to run and because running makes us high (runners high of course). But many run for the fitness and health benefits. Hundreds of studies have been conducted on the health benefits of running over the past 50 years from Stanford to Harvard and published in prestigious medical journals. The following is a brief run-down of the health benefits of running:

1. **Cardiovascular Health:** Running as little as 5-10 minutes per day has shown to increase life span by several years. Running can reduce triglycerides and bad cholesterol while raising good cholesterol. Running has been shown to reduce blood pressure and resting heart rate and improve circulation throughout the body. It makes the heart stronger and more efficient, and improves the way oxygen is utilized.

2. **Stress Relief:** One of my favorite benefits of running is the "runner's high". Running induces the release of endorphins and increases dopamine levels which creates a feeling of euphoria and relaxation and naturally relieves stress.

3. **Weight Loss:** Any endurance exercise will increase aerobic capacity and rev up the body's metabolism to burn fat, but running is the king of the hill (and running hills will jack up your fat burning even more) of burning calories if it's done correctly. Books and articles abound on the topic of running methods but I've found my routine has worked well:

   • High Intensity Interval Training (HIIT): Numerous studies have proven this method is the best for burning fat and increasing overall health and fitness. There are many theories on HIIT but I simply run at a comfortable pace for 3 minutes...then increase my pace and run as fast as I can for 30 – 60 seconds...followed by 3 minutes at a comfortable pace and repeat this for 20 – 30 minutes. HIIT conditions the body to utilize oxygen more efficiently and improves the hearts' ability to pump while increasing the body's metabolism. And studies show that metabolism stays high long after a HIIT run so fat burning takes place long after you've unlaced your running shoes.

   • Endurance Run: Some call this a long run but "long" can be defined differently by different people. To some, a long run may be 25 or 30 miles (100 miles for the crazy, yet incredibly fit ultra-runners), but for many of us a long run is 5 or 10 miles. The endurance run is designed to keep the heart rate elevated at a steady rate over a prolonged period of time. This run will burn calories during the run but doesn't boost the metabolism (fat burning while sedentary) as much as HIIT. The endurance run is a necessary component of weight loss and overall fitness.

4. **Long Life**: According to a large-scale study of exercise and mortality, running for as little as five minutes a day could significantly lower a person's risk of dying prematurely. The findings suggest the benefits of even small amounts of vigorous exercise may be much greater than experts had assumed. In recent years, moderate exercise, such as brisk walking, has been the focus of a great deal of exercise science and most exercise recommendations. The government's formal exercise guidelines, for instance, suggest people should engage in about 30 minutes of moderate exercise on most days of the week.

But a study, published in The Journal of the American College of Cardiology, proves moderate exercise may not provide optimum benefit. Researchers from Iowa State University and the University of South Carolina turned to a huge database maintained at the Cooper Clinic and Cooper Institute in Dallas.

For decades, researchers there have been collecting information about the health of tens of thousands of men and women visiting the clinic for check-ups. These adults, after completing extensive medical and fitness examinations, have filled out questionnaires about their exercise habits, including whether, how often and how fast they ran.

From this database, the researchers chose the records of 55,137 healthy men and women ages 18 to 100 who had visited the clinic at least 15 years before the start of the study. Of this group, 24% identified themselves as runners, although their typical mileage and pace varied greatly. The researchers then checked death records for these adults. In 15 years almost 3,500 had died, many from heart disease. But the runners were much less susceptible than the non-runners. The runners' risk of dying from any cause was 30 percent lower than that for the non-runners, and their risk of dying from heart disease was 45 percent lower, even when the researchers adjusted for being overweight or for smoking. And even overweight smokers who ran were less likely to die prematurely than people who did not run. As a group, runners gained two - three extra years of life compared with those adults who never ran.

Action Plan: The dose of running for optimum results vary. As little as 5-10 minutes per day have been shown to have a profound benefit on health, while running marathons has been shown to be very hard on the body. I believe the right dose depends on several factors including fitness levels and goals. For me the right dose is 25-45 minutes per day, alternating interval runs (speed) and longer runs.

From Dr. Blair's Blog

CBD & Weight Loss

Ever wonder why cannabis users get the "munchies" but rarely get fat? I did, so I looked into it and found that a cannabinoid in cannabis called CBD is responsible for keeping the fat off!

In research published late last year, scientists from the University of Miami reported that regular cannabis users were 54% less likely to suffer from metabolic syndrome than their non-using counterparts. According to the Mayo Clinic, metabolic syndrome is a term for a series of co-occurring health conditions that include:

- High blood pressure
- High blood sugar
- Excess body fat around the waist and belly

When these factors all occur together, they increase your likelihood of developing diabetes and heart disease.

The study examined data from nearly 8,500 individuals through National Health and Nutrition Surveys. Participants were between the 20 and 59-years-old and they found cannabis users on average:

- Had lower blood sugar levels
- Less risk of developing type 2 Diabetes
- Less abdominal fat
- Reduced risk of heart disease
- Lower levels of bad cholesterol.

These findings are in tune with other research on marijuana and metabolism. Research from 2013 and 2014 has shown that regular cannabis have lower BMIs smaller waistlines: up to 1.5 inches smaller than non-users. In the face of a worldwide obesity epidemic, the scientific community is struggling to figure out just how cannabis is able to have such a positive effect on metabolism.

Researchers at the School of Pharmacy in Berkshire's University treated male rats with three different cannabinoids and watched to see how each chemical affected the rodents' appetite. The three cannabinoids they tested were:

- cannabigerol (CBG)
- cannabinol (CBN)
- cannabidiol (CBD)

They found that CBN caused rats to eat more while CBG had no effect on their appetites. But, CBD worked like magic. The rats still ate, but their overall food intake was less during the test period. These findings on CBD confirm what a handful of other studies have also shown.

In 2012, scientists in Budapest found that CBD was effective at reducing the amount of fat build-up inside arteries caused by a high sugar diet. A study from 2011 found that CBD protected insulin-producing cells from damage in the pancreas. Another study from 2010 found that CBD decreased the body weight of adult rats.

The research is clear that CBD from cannabis can have a positive impact on body weight and metabolic syndrome.

Stories of Healing
"I Have a Crushing Headache"

I have been studying and practicing nutrition and herbal medicine for over 25 years and have been fortunate enough to have counselled hundreds of people over those years. I have been able to recommend natural treatments to help people with everything from ADHD to weight loss, and everything in between, but when you're living with the person dealing with issues it takes on a whole new urgency.

I married my wife Patty in May of 2014 at a beautiful, 250 year old church in our hometown. Together, we have 4 beautiful girls, 2 large dogs, and a lizard. Okay, the lizard is mine and though Patty and the girls pretend to be aggravated to have a pet lizard in the house, they really do like him! So, with a cool new husband, 4 teenagers, 2 dogs, a lizard, and a demanding career it's easy to see why Patty would have an occasional headache. Unfortunately, the occasional headache became more and more common and progressively worse until she told me one day, *"I have a crushing headache"*! These crushing headaches became more frequent and she took more over-the-counter pain medication that usually did not help much.

I knew that a component of cannabis that is legal in North Carolina called CBD oil could help alleviate Patty's severe tension headaches but I knew if I told her what it was she would have doubts about taking it. So I found a peppermint flavored CBD oil and simply told her to take 2 sprays of this "peppermint oil" every morning to see if it would help with the headaches. As expected, the CBD oil did help alleviate the headaches, reducing both the frequency and severity of them. CBD (cannabadiol) is a powerful medicine to fight inflammation and pain throughout the body. Oh, and I finally told Patty what the "peppermint spray" was and she continues to take it as a preventative.

"I Don't Want to Have a Hysterectomy"

One of the most prevalent topics I am asked to discuss in consultations has to do with hormones. After all, hormones run the whole show and if they get out of balance it can affect how we live from day-to-day. Gerri came to me with excruciating menstrual pain, often keeping her bed-ridden several days each month. She had consulted with her doctor who just kept prescribing powerful narcotic pain medicines at higher and higher doses. These powerful pain meds became more ineffective and she found a doctor willing to do something more than just prescribe a pain pill to cover up the symptoms.

Gerri's doctor scheduled exploratory surgery to determine the source of the horrible menstrual pain. She was then diagnosed with endometriosis and told she had two options. **Just two!** She could be prescribed a new drug that would put her in menopause (at 34 years-of-age), or she could have a hysterectomy. That's it…**two** choices! Neither choice was acceptable to Gerri, who told me that at 34 she didn't want menopause **or** hysterectomy!

Her doctors had not even bothered to address any underlying reason or cause of the endometriosis. They only wanted to give her a prescription or do surgery and send her on her way. During our consultation I explained how years of hormone imbalance and estrogen-dominance had caused the endometriosis. Gerri began taking the herbs I recommended and within 3 months the pain was gone! She took:

- **Vitex (Chaste Berry) to balance progesterone & estrogen**
- **Indole 3 Carbinol (I3C) & DIM to metabolize excess estrogen**
- **Systemic Proteolytic Enzymes to break up scar tissues**
- **An adaptogenic blend containing ashwagandha to reduce stress hormones and strengthen adrenal gland function.**

Gerri continues taking the herbs I recommended and remains pain-free many years later.

"I Can't Breathe Walking to the Mailbox"
Roger's wife Linda came to me to discuss her husband's COPD and emphysema because he was too tired to leave the house. Linda told me

that Roger, a veteran of the Korean War, is on oxygen and rarely leaves home. She said that he can't even walk to the mailbox most days without losing his breath.

Roger's doctors at the VA had done all they knew to do for him. Linda told me that they had tried antibiotics, steroids, inhalers, and now he walks around dragging an oxygen tank. Linda wanted to know if there were any natural treatments he could try.

I told Linda that Robert should remove things from his diet that cause inflammation, such as canola oils and sugar, and take curcumin and fish oil to help reduce inflammation. I also told Linda about the remarkable healing power of liquid, green chlorophyll.

Chlorophyll is the "life blood" of plants and has a proven ability to cleanse the lungs as well as improve lung function, including improving the lung's ability to utilize oxygen. I told Linda to discuss this plan with Roger's doctor before getting started and she did. She reported back to me that his doctor told them, "I don't believe in untested, herbal hoaxes but it probably isn't harmful so go ahead".

So after several years of blindly following his doctor's advice and taking prescriptions that barely masked the symptoms, Roger began the journey of regaining his health. He took curcumin, fish oil, and chlorophyll every day while reducing the consumption of sugar and vegetable oils.

Three months after my initial visit with Linda, Robert and Linda came to see me. Robert told me that he was amazed that he is no longer on oxygen, and not only can he walk to the mailbox now...he's taking walks with Linda around the neighborhood!

Our bodies desire to be healthy and have a remarkable ability to heal if given the proper nutrients.

A New Blog Entry:

The Amazing Benefits of Berberine

Berberine is a yellow alkaloid found in the roots of several plants including goldenseal. It has been used in Traditional Chinese Medicine for several thousand years and modern research is confirming that this is a powerful healing herb. It has been proven to be anti-bacterial, anti-viral, and anti-fungal as well as a potent regulator of blood sugar and triglycerides. Berberine is one of the few herbs that can increase the cellular activity of AMPK, an enzyme that regulates cell health and longevity as well as fat metabolism. Here is what the research shows:

Berberine & Blood Sugar

Type 2 diabetes is a serious disease that has become way too common in recent decades, causing millions of deaths every year. It is characterized by elevated blood sugar (glucose) levels, either caused by insulin resistance or lack of insulin. Over time, high blood sugar levels can damage the body's tissues and organs, leading to various health problems and a shortened lifespan. Many studies show that berberine can significantly reduce blood sugar levels in individuals with type 2 diabetes.

Its effectiveness is comparable to the popular diabetes drug metformin (Jun Yin 2008) and seems to work through multiple different actions:

- **Decreases insulin resistance, making the blood sugar lowering hormone insulin more effective.**
- **Increases glycolysis, helping the body break down sugars inside cells.**
- **Decreases sugar production in the liver.**
- **Slows the breakdown of carbohydrates in the digestive tract.**

- In one study of 116 diabetic patients, 1000 mg of berberine per day lowered fasting blood sugar by 20%. It also lowered hemoglobin A1C by 12% (a marker for long-term blood sugar levels), and also lowered blood lipids like cholesterol and triglycerides (J Clin Endocrinol Metab. 2008 Jul;93(7):2559-65).

Berberine & Weight Loss

- In a 12-week study in overweight individuals, participants took 500 mg three times per day. Those in the study lost an average of 5 pounds. The participants also lost 3.6% of their body fat (Jing Yang,2012).
- Another study was conducted with 37 men and women with metabolic syndrome. This study lasted 3 months, and the participants took 300 mg, 3 times per day. The participants dropped their body mass index (BMI) levels from 31.5 to 27.4 in only 3 months. They also lost belly fat and improved many health markers such as blood sugar and triglycerides.

The researchers believe that the weight loss is caused by improved function of fat-regulating hormones, such as insulin, leptin, and AMPK.

6

The Herb Doctor's Medicine Chest

I have been studying herbal medicine from villages around the world for nearly 30 years. Our bodies were designed to utilize herbs and food for medicine and herbs have been considered medicine for thousands of years. Prescription drugs can only mask symptoms of disease but herbs and food (herbs are food) give the body the nutrients it needs to heal itself. The human body has a remarkable ability to heal if given the tools it needs.

Here is a list of herbs that I think everyone should know. I'll list each herb's name, origin, historic use, and modern usage:

Alfalfa
Scientific Name: Medicago sativa
Common Names: Buffalo grass
Part Used: Leaves, stems, sprouts
Habitat: Alfalfa is native to southwestern Asia and Southeastern Europe. Also grows in North America and North Africa.

Alfalfa is loaded with important vitamins, minerals, trace minerals and protein. Its roots go down as far as 30 feet to pull valuable nutrients from the earth. This plant is commonly used for arthritis, digestive problems, as a diuretic, and for reducing high cholesterol. It's a source of easily digested nutrients. Alfalfa is high in beta-carotene and builds the immune system. This plant also contains chlorophyll, which is good for lung health as well as reducing bad breath and body odor.

Aloe
Scientific Name: Aloe vera
Common Names: Aloe, cape
Part Used: Leaves
Habitat: Aloe is native to the Mediterranean. It also grows in Latin America and the Caribbean.

The gel inside of the leaves of the Aloe plant can be used externally to treat minor burns, sun burn, cuts, scrapes and poison ivy. Aloe gel is good for moisturizing the skin and is a main ingredient of many skin care products. Many people use it to reduce acne and treat other skin problems.

American Ginseng
Scientific Name: Panax quinquefolius
Common Names: Ginseng, xi yang shen
Part Used: Root
Habitat: American Ginseng grows in the eastern part of North America and Canada.

American ginseng is an adaptogen. An adaptogen is a substance which protects against stress of all types. This type of ginseng has been used to strengthen the immune system, increase strength and stamina, treat digestive disorders, treat diabetes, treat ADHD and as a general tonic for wellnes. American ginseng is considered a cooling ginseng, where Korean ginseng has a more warming effect on the body.

Amla
Scientific Name: Phyllanthus emblica
Common Names: Indian gooseberry
Part Used: Fruit
Habitat: Amla is native to India

Amla is used in the Ayurvedic medicine system of India. It is rich in vitamin C and contains many vitamins, minerals and antioxidants. Amla is used to treat inflammation of the joints, fevers, urinary tract infections and to control blood sugar. It is high in fiber and may be helpful in treating constipation.

Arnica
Scientific Name: Arnica montana
Common Names: Leopard's bane, mountain daisy, mountain arnica
Part Used: Flowers
Habitat: Arnica is native to central Asia, Siberia and Europe.

Arnica is used externally as an ointment for sore muscles, sprains and bruises. It possesses anti-inflammatory, analgesic and anti-septic properties.

Ashwagandha
Scientific Name: Withania Somnifera
Part Used: Roots
Habitat: Ashwagandha grows in India, Africa and widely cultivated around the world

Ashwagandha is considered a powerful adaptogen. This means that is has a beneficial normalizing effect on the entire body.

Ashwagandha is often used as a rejuvenator. It can also be used as a sedative, anti-inflammatory, diuretic, and to increase physical energy and endurance

In India, Ashwaganda is often prescribed to elderly patients for the treatment of cerebral disorders, such as memory loss. Some research suggests that this herb can increase acetylcholine receptor activity, partially explaining its benefit to the brain. It has been used historically for increasing cognitive ability.

Researchers at the University of Texas found that extracts of Ashwaganda had similar effects on the brain as the nutrient GABA, making it good for reducing anxiety.

Taking Ashwagandha can calm the mind, promoting better more restful sleep. It does this by calming the nerves and improving a person's ability to handle physical and emotional stress.

Ashwagandha has anti-inflammatory action and is often taken to treat rheumatoid arthritis. There is a naturally occurring steroid in the herb that is similar to hydrocortisone. Its pain relieving action is as effective as aspirin.

Ashwagandha is popular with athletes. It can promote better oxygen flow the muscles, helping to increase strength and endurance during exercise. This would enable the athlete to gain more lean muscle than normally possible. It can also reduce the effect of stress hormones and reduce lactic acid build-up.

Astragalus
Scientific Name: Astragalus membranaceus
Common Names: Huang qi
Part Used: Roots
Habitat: Astragalus is native to Mongolia and China.

Astragalus is one of the most popular herbs in the traditional Chinese medicine system. It has been in use for over 3000 years. This herb is most often used as a diuretic and for lowering high blood pressure. Many people use it to treat upper respiratory infections as well as the common cold, as it seems to increase the production of white blood cells. Traditionally, astragalus has also been used to increase energy, strengthen the immune system, treat excessive sweating, ulcers and diarrhea.

Bacopa
Scientific Name: Bacopa Monnieri
Common Names: Brahmi, Water hyssop
Part Used: Whole plant.
Habitat: Bacopa is native to India

Bacopa has been used as an effective brain tonic in the Ayurvedic system of medicine for 3000 years in India. It is beneficial to long and short term memory. The plant's saponins have a positive effect on the brain's neurotransmitters. Bacopa is now being studied as a possible treatment for ADHD, Alzheimer's and Parkinson's disease. Bacopa is often used to treat depression, anxiety asthma, allergies and bronchitis. It also has some anti-inflammatory properties.

Bilberry
Scientific Name: Vaccinium mytillus
Common Names: European blueberry, huckleberry
Part Used: Leaves, fruits
Habitat: Bilberry grows in the warm regions of the Northern Hemisphere

Bilberry is most often used to prevent night blindness. It seems to be able to strengthen the capillaries and protect them from free radical damage. This plant contains flavonoids (antioxidants)called anthocyanosides.

Black Cherry
Scientific Name: Prunus serotina
Common Names: Bird cherry, rum cherry

Part Used: Bark
Habitat: Black Cherry is native to North America

Native Americans used black cherry as a medicinal herb to treat coughs. The bark from the black cherry tree was often made into a tea or syrup and used to expel worms, heal ulcers and treat burns. They also used it as a remedy for sore throat, pneumonia and lack of appetite. Black Cherry bark contains a glycoside called prunasin which quells spasms in the smooth muscles of the bronchioles.

Black Cohosh
Scientific Name: Cimicifuga racemosa
Common Names: Black snakeroot, bugwort
Part Used: Roots, rhizome
Habitat: Black Cohosh is native to North America

The Cherokee Indians used black cohosh as a diuretic and as a remedy for fatigue and tuberculosis. Others have used this herb to treat menstrual irregularities, rheumatism and sore throat. Today, black cohosh is used mainly to reduce the severity of premenopausal and menopausal symptoms, such as excessive sweating, depression and hot flashes.

Boneset
Scientific Name: Eupatorium perfoliatum
Common Names: Indian sage, feverwort
Part Used: Leaves and flowers
Habitat: Boneset is native to North America

Boneset was used by the Native Americans to induce sweating and to treat colds, flu, arthritis, indigestion, loss of appetite, and constipation. This plant is still in use today to treat colds, flu, fever and minor inflammation.

Borage
Scientific Name: Borago officinalis
Common Names: star flower, bee Plant
Part Used: Flowers, seed oil
Habitat: Borage is native to Southern Europe

Borage is often used to treat fever, lung infections, inflammation, and as a diuretic. It may also be effective as a mild anti-depressant and sedative. Oil from Borage seeds are a rich source of gammalinolenic acid (GLA). GLA is a fatty acid used by the body to boost immunity and fight inflammation.

Boswellia
Scientific Name: Boswellia serrata
Common Names: Indian frankincense, guggul
Part Used: Resin
Habitat: Boswellia is native to Africa and Asia

Boswellia has been used in the Ayurvedic medicine system of India for over 3,000 years. Ancient healers used it to treat conditions such as asthma, fevers, cardiovascular disorders, rheumatism, and diabetes. Today, this herb is mostly used to treat inflammation and pain of the joints.

A more modern use of boswellia is for treating inflammation. The boswellic acid that comes from the tree's resin and sap acts as a 5-LOX (5-lipoxygenase) inhibitor and is used to treat rheumatoid and osteoarthritis, asthma, menstrual cramps and inflammatory bowel disease.

Buchu
Scientific Name: Agathosma betulina
Common Names: bucco, bookoo
Part Used: Leaves
Habitat: Buchu is native to South Africa

Buchu is most often used as a stimulating tonic and a diuretic. It is now commonly used to treat urinary tract infections. In the past, this herb has also been used to treat arthritis, kidney stones and gout.

Burdock
Scientific Name: Arctium Lappa
Common Names: Wild Burdock, beggar's buttons
Part Used: Seeds, leaves and roots
Habitat: Burdock grows in the United States, Europe, Japan and China

Burdock was used by the ancient Greeks to treat wounds and infections. This herb is often used to treat liver and digestive problems, urinary tract infections, ulcers, eczema, psoriasis and to boost energy and stamina. It has anti-fungal and anti-bacterial properties and makes a good immune system booster and blood purifier.

Butterbur
Scientific Name: Petasites hybridus
Common Names: Common butterbur, coughwort
Part Used: Leaves, rhizomes
Habitat: Butterbur is native to Asia and Europe

Butterbur has traditionally been used to treat coughs, urinary problems, fever and parasites. Now this herb is mostly used as an anti-inflammatory agent and to treat migraine headaches. It is sometimes used to reduce smooth muscle spasms. Some studies have found butterbur effective in reducing bronchial spasms in people having bronchitis and asthma.

Calendula
Scientific Name: Calendula officinalis
Common Names: Pot marigold

Part Used: Flowers
Habitat: Calendula is native to the Mediterranean region

Historically, calendula was used to induce menstruation, break fevers, cure jaundice, treat open sores and for liver and stomach problems. It has antiseptic and anti-inflammatory properties and can be used externally for sunburn and eczema. Today this herb is most often used externally to treat slow healing wounds and to promote tissue repair.

Cascara Sagrada
Scientific Name: Frangula purshiana
Common Names: Cascara buckthron, sacred bark
Part Used: Bark
Habitat: Cascara Sagrada is native to the Pacific Northwest in North America

Cascara Sagrada was used by Native Americans as a laxative and to treat constipation, colitis, upset stomach, jaundice and hemorrhoids. Today it is sometimes used as a laxative.

Cat's Claw
Scientific Name: Uncaria tomentosa
Common Names: Peruvian cat's claw
Part Used: Bark, root
Habitat: Cat's Claw is native to South and Central America

Cat's claw has been used by the natives of Peru for several thousand years to treat conditions such as asthma, arthritis, urinary tract infections, ulcers and intestinal problems. Today, this herb is most often used to boost the immune system and as an anti-inflammatory.

Cayenne
Scientific Name: Capsicum annuum
Common Names: Red pepper, capsicum, chili pepper
Part Used: Fruit
Habitat: Cayenne is native to tropical regions of the Americas

Cayenne was used by Native Americans as a pain reliever and infections. It was also used for toothache, arthritis and to aid digestion. This herb has anti-bacterial properties, can stimulate blood flow and is rich in antioxidants. Many people consume cayenne to maintain cardiovascular health as studies suggest that it may be able to reduce triglyceride levels and platelet aggregation in the blood.

Chamomile
Scientific Name: Matricaria recutita
Common Names: German chamomile, wild chamomile
Part Used: Flower heads, oil
Habitat: Chamomile is native to Asia, Africa and Europe

Used by the ancient Egyptians for fever and chills, chamomile is still in wide use today. This plant is used for colic, indigestion, flatulence, bloating heartburn and to calm nervousness.

Chaste Tree (Vitex)
Scientific Name: Vitex agnus-castus
Common Names: Chaste berry, vitex
Part Used: Fruits
Habitat: The chaste tree is native to Southern Europe and Western Asia

For over 2,000 years the chaste tree (Vitex) has been used to treat gynecological problems such as relieving menstrual cramps, promoting normal menstruation and to balance hormones.

Cinnamon
Scientific Name: Cinnamonum verum
Common Names: Chinese cassia, ceylon cinnamon
Part Used: Bark
Habitat: Cinnamon is native to India. Cultivated in Indonesia, Africa and South America.

Cinnamon is most often used to soothe digestion, treat colds, nausea and inflammation. Cinnamon's essential oil has antifungal, antibacterial and antispasmodic properties and is useful in regulating blood sugar.

Cordyceps
Scientific Name: Cordyceps sinensis
Common Names: Caterpillar fungus, Zhiling
Part Used: Fruiting body
Habitat: Cordyceps mushrooms grows wild in the Himalayan Mountains

This mushroom has a long history of use in Chinese herbalism. It is considered a great tonic for building physical strength and endurance. Cordyceps dilates the lung's airways allowing more oxygen to reach the blood. For this fact it is very popular with athletes. This healing mushroom is also used to treat asthma, cough and bronchitis. It possesses anti-inflammatory properties and has the ability to relax the bronchial walls and is a great immune system booster.

It has been used in the past to strengthen the immune system by increasing the amount of the body's natural killer cells. It benefits the entire vascular system by regulating blood pressure, strengthening the muscles of the heart and improving circulation. It protects the kidney and liver by improving blood flow.

Cordyceps is used by athletes to improve endurance and performance. The Chinese Olympic athletes are known to consume it while training and competing and is said to noticeably increase the physical strength and stamina of anyone who consumes it.

Dandelion
Scientific Name: Taraxacum officinale
Common Names: Lion's tooth
Part Used: Leaves, flowers, root
Habitat: Dandelion is native to Europe and Asia but grow all over the world

The dandelion has been used for thousands of years for its medicinal properties. It is used as a potent diuretic and detoxifying herb. Other common uses of this plant were to treat breast inflammation, digestive disorders, and appendicitis.

Dong Quai
Scientific Name: Angelica sinensis
Common Names: Chinese angelica
Part Used: Root
Habitat: This herb is native to China, Japan, and Korea

Dong Quai is used as a remedy for menstrual cycle disorder and to treat symptoms such as bleeding of the uterus and menstruation pain. It is helpful for relieving vaginal dryness, hot flashes, mood swings and PMS.

Echinacea
Scientific Name: Echinacea purpurea
Common Names: Purple coneflower
Part Used: Roots, leaves and flowers
Habitat: Echinacea is native to Central and Eastern North America

Echinacea is very popular for treating colds and flu. This herb is a great immune system booster. It can treat sore throat and upper respiratory tract infections. It is a good detoxifier and has antiviral, anti-inflammatory and antibiotic properties.

Fo-Ti
Scientific Name: Polygonum Multiflorum
Common Names: He Shou Wu, climbing knotweed
Part Used: Root
Habitat: Fo-Ti is native to China

Fo-Ti is a famous longevity herb that has been in constant use in China for 3000 years. It is very popular with older men and is said to be able to turn one's hair back to its youthful color and appearance. It is a powerful adaptogen herb for strength and vitality.

Ginkgo Biloba
Scientific Name: Ginkgo biloba
Common Names: Ginkgo
Part Used: Leaves and seeds
Habitat: Ginkgo biloba is native China but is also cultivated in Japan, France and the southern United States.

Ginkgo Biloba improves the flow of blood to the brain and increases oxygen to the brain cells. It is often used as an effective cognitive enhancer and memory booster.

Ginkgo possesses anti-coagulating properties and prevents the formation of blood clots. This could in turn reduce risk of stroke. This herb contains powerful antioxidants. Its flavonoids protect the body from free radical damage and cell oxidation.

Gynostemma (Jiaogulan)
Scientific Name: Gynostemma Pentaphyllum
Common Names: Jiaogulan, southern ginseng, Xianao
Part Used: Leaves
Habitat: Gynostemma is native to China, Korea, Vietnam, Taiwan

Gynostema or "Jiaogulan" is an adaptogenic herb. It increases strength and stamina and protects the body and mind against stress, both mental and physical. It is especially helpful for the immune, digestive, nervous, reproductive, and cardiovascular systems.

Gynostemma is used to reduce fatigue, treat bronchitis, improve sexual function and to strengthen the body in general and is considered a very powerful tonic for wellbeing.

Gynostemma is also capable of lowering bad cholesterol (LDL) and triglycerides while increasing good cholesterol (HDL). It can lower high blood pressure and improve cardio-vascular health by increasing coronary blood flow and decreasing vascular resistance. It enhances the production of nitric oxide which relaxes the blood vessels.

Gynostemma can increase the antioxidant superoxide dismutase (SOD). SOD prevents oxidation damage from harmful free radicals. Jiaogulan is very popular with athletes because of its strength and endurance enhancing properties.

Holy Basil
Scientific Name: Ocimum Sanctum
Common Names: Tulsi
Part Used: Leaves, Stems
Habitat: Holy Basil is native to India

Holy Basil is used for reducing stress, anxiety and depression. It is also known to enhance cerebral circulation and improve memory.

Kava

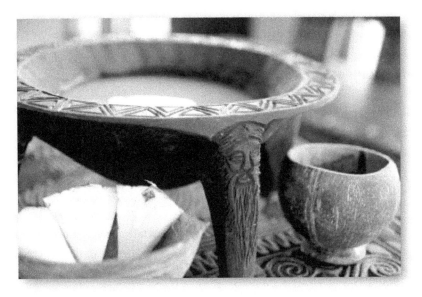

Scientific Name: Piper Methysticum
Common Names: Awa
Part Used: Rhizome, roots
Habitat: Kava grows on the Pacific Islands

Villagers of the South Pacific Islands have consumed kava for over 3000 years to relax at the end of a day and in tribal ceremonies. It is used to quell arguments and make important decisions. It is said that it is impossible to hate with kava in you.

Kavalactones are responsible for kava's relaxing effect and are found in the root of the plant. Kava is a member of the pepper family and its name piper methysticum translates to "intoxicating pepper". Kava also has a mild analgesic effect causing a pleasant numbness in the mouth for a few minutes after consuming it.

Kava has a very calming effect on the mind and muscles and can be slightly intoxicating, yet different than alcohol in that it does not affect motor skills or ability to function (drive a car, etc). Several studies from Duke University and Maryland University have shown that kava is a safe alternative to prescription benzodiazepines for anxiety. Kava is instantly relaxing when consumed and is known as "the **root** of happiness".

Lemongrass
Scientific Name: Cymbopogon citratus
Common Names: Silky heads, fever grass
Part Used: Grass
Habitat: Lemongrass is native to tropical Asia and India

Lemongrass tea is a relaxing beverage that helps reduce anxiety and promote sound sleep. Used externally, it can treat skin conditions.

Licorice Root
Scientific Name: Glycyrrhiza Uralensis
Common Names: Guo Lao, sweat herb, sweet wood, beauty grass, elf grass, pink grass
Part Used: Root
Habitat: Licorice root is native to Asia

Licorice root is a very popular herb in Chinese medicine. It is a powerful adrenal tonic to balance hormones and is a digestive aid.

Lycium Fruit (Goji)
Scientific Name: Lycium barbarum
Common Names: Goji, wolfberry
Part Used: Fruit
Habitat: Lycium grows in Northwestern China and Tibet

Goji fruit has been consumed for centuries in China for its sweet taste and health giving properties. The berries from the

Lycium plant are one of the most nutritious foods on earth and contain a very high level of antioxidants.

Maca
Scientific Name: Lepidium meyenii
Common Names: Peruvian ginseng
Part Used: Root
Habitat: Maca is native to Peru

Maca is an adaptogen that helps the body cope with stress. This root is rich in vitamins, minerals, plant sterols and amino acids. Inca people refer to it as a "superfood". Studies have found that consuming maca root can greatly enhance physical strength and stamina as well as boost the libido. It's a great overall energy booster and is popular with athletes. Maca is beneficial to the nervous system and is calming to the nerves. Today, this herb is mostly used for increasing energy and balancing the sex hormones.

Milk Thistle
Scientific Name: Silybum marianum
Common Names: Silymarin, Mary Thistle
Part Used: Seeds
Habitat: Milk Thistle is native to Europe

Milk thistle seeds contain silymarin which can protect and detoxify the liver.

Neem
Scientific Name: Azadirachta indica
Part Used: Leaf, Bark, Oil
Habitat: Neem trees grow in India

The neem tree grows throughout India and has been used as medicine both internally and externally for over 2000 years. It is considered "the village pharmacy" in India because it can help treat so many conditions. The leaf is used internally to fight infection, reduce fever, and balance blood sugar. The bark of the tree can be used externally as an insect repellent and the oil is used to heal skin conditions.

Rhodiola
Scientific Name: Rhodiola Rosea
Common Names: Golden Root, Arctic Root, Aaron's Rod
Part Used: Root
Habitat: Rhodiola is native Siberia

Rhodiola rosea is very popular with Russian athletes due to its ability to enhance physical strength and endurance. Besides its beneficial effects on the body, this herb is often used to keep the mind sharp and improve memory. It is now gaining popularity as a natural anti-depressant. Rhodiola is considered an adaptogen, protecting the body from the damaging effects of stress.

Saw Palmetto
Scientific Name: Serenoa repens
Common Names: palmetto berry
Part Used: Fruit
Habitat: Saw Palmetto grows in the islands of the West Indies and Southeastern United States

Saw Palmetto is often used to treat Benign Prostatic Hyperplasia (BPH) and its symptoms, like the need to urinate frequently. Another popular use of this herb is to treat male pattern baldness by reducing the body's levels of dihydrotestosterone (DHT).

Schizandra
Scientific Name: Schizandra chinensis
Common Names: Schisandra, Five flavor berry, Wu wei zi,

Part Used: Fruit
Habitat: Schizandra is native to northern China

Schizandra berries have been consumed throughout China for several thousand years to improve strength and endurance as well as reduce stress. Chinese athletes have incorporated schizandra into their training and research proves it can provide energy before a workout and help in recovery after.

Shilajit

Scientific Name: Asphaltum
Common Names: Mineral Pitch
Part Used: The resin
Habitat: Shilajit can be found in the Himalayan Mountains of Nepal and Tibet.

Shilajit is loaded with vitamins and minerals and has been consumed in India for centuries to increase energy and adapt to stress. It can boost the sex hormones and rejuvenate the body.

Shilajit is considered one of the most important substances in the Indian system of Ayurvedic medicine. Its name means "nectar of God".

Shilajit is a thick, blackish-brown mineral pitch resin that oozes out of cracks in the Himalayan mountains as the summer heat raises the temperature of the rock and is composed of centuries old, decomposed plants which are a potent source of vitamins, minerals and other nutrients. It is nature's most potent trace mineral source. It's a powerful adaptogen, helping protect against all types of mental and physical stress.

Siberian Ginseng (Eleuthero)

Scientific Name: Eleutherococcus senticosus
Common Names: Siberian ginseng, eleuthero
Part Used: Root

Habitat: Siberian Ginseng is native to Russia, China and Korea

Siberian ginseng (Eleuthero) is considered an energizer and stress reducer. It has been used for hundreds of years as an invigorating tonic herb. It is a powerful adaptogen that can normalize the body and bring it back into balance.

Skullcap
Scientific Name: Scutellaria lateriflora
Common Names: quaker bonnet
Part Used: The whole plant
Habitat: Skullcap grows in Europe, Asia, Canada and the United States

Skullcap is an ancient sleep aid. It can greatly reduce anxiety and nervousness and is often called nature's tranquilizer. Many people take it to relieve muscle spasms and twitches and lower blood pressure. Skullcap also possesses anti-inflammatory properties and may be useful for treating arthritis and joint pain.

St. John's Wort
Scientific Name: Hypericum perforatum
Common Names: goat weed
Part Used: Flower
Habitat: St. John's Wort grows in Europe, The United States and Australia

St. John's Wort is known as Nature's anti-depressant. It is often used to treat depression and anxiety. It functions as an SSRI (selective serotonin reuptake inhibitor). This allows more serotonin to stay where it's needed to keep you feeling less depressed and anxious. This herb is also used to help quit smoking. St. John's work possesses antiviral properties and can be used externally to treat wounds.

Turmeric

Scientific Name: Curcuma longa
Part Used: Root
Habitat: Turmeric is native to India

Turmeric has been used in India for over 3000 years and is a major part of the Ayurvedic system of medicine. It was first used as a dye and then later for its medicinal properties.

The powerful antioxidant curcumin is the active ingredient in turmeric and is what gives it its golden color.

Turmeric is a great natural liver detoxifier. Studies conducted at The University of Maryland Medical Center suggest that it works as an antioxidant, protecting the liver against damage by free radicals and helps increase the production of bile by the gallbladder. It is often used in the treatment of gallstones and liver disorders by the systems of Chinese and Ayurvedic medicine.

Turmeric is also very effective as a pain reliever and inflammation reducer. Research suggests that the curcumin in turmeric inhibits the production of COX-2, an enzyme in the body that causes inflammation. It works just as well as many prescription anti-inflammatory medicines, but without the negative side-effects.

This herb possesses antibiotic and antiseptic properties. It can be used for disinfecting cuts, scrapes and burns. It aids in fat metabolism and may be helpful for people trying to lose weight. The Chinese have long used turmeric as an effective treatment for depression.

Valerian Root

Scientific Name: Valerian officinalis
Common Names: St. George's Herb
Part Used: Root

Habitat: Valerian is native to Western Europe, Asia and North America

Valerian is an ancient remedy for insomnia and a great stress buster. Many people find it an effective treatment for anxiety as well. The active components of this herb help increase the production of gamma amino butyric acid (GABA). The brain needs GABA to sleep deeper and relax.

7

"Whacky" Things I Do For Health

(that make Patty roll her eyes at me)

Oil Pulling

Oil pulling, also known as "kavala" or "gundusha," is an ancient Ayurvedic dental technique that involves swishing a tablespoon of oil in your mouth on an empty stomach for around 20 minutes. This action reportedly draws out toxins in your body, primarily to improve oral health but also to improve your overall health.

A study published in Journal of Indian Society of Preventive Dentistry (2008) showed that oil pulling with sesame oil can boost overall oral health by significantly reducing Streptococcus mutans, a microbe that contributes to tooth decay. Researchers believe the lipids in the oil reduce the adhesion of bacteria to the teeth and gums, possibly explaining its bacteria-diminishing effects.

Other research shows that oil pulling can relieve bad breath. This same research has also shown that oil pulling can noticeably reduce the presence of plaque to support the health of teeth and gums (Journal of Indian Society of Preventive Dentistry (2011). Research also shows that swishing with sesame oil produces a saponification process, or a process in which the oil produces a soap-like effect in the mouth, insuring that the oil reaches deep into hard to reach places.

Some studies prove that cavities have been shown to be reduced by up to 50% in persons who practice oil pulling (African Journal of Microbiology Research Vol.(2) 2008). The oil used in this study was sesame oil; perhaps one of the most popular oils used in oil pulling, and showed very powerful activity in the mouth. Just 40 days of oil pulling resulted in a 20% decrease in oral bacteria.

Traditional benefits beyond dental health:

Traditional Ayurvedic practitioners cite other benefits of oil pulling. It is believed that oil pulling stimulates the lymphatic system and aids in the transport of toxins away from vital organs. The reported benefits of oil pulling include:

- **Teeth whitening**
- **Clearer skin**
- **Improved digestion**
- **Weight loss**
- **Normal sleep patterns**
- **Improved kidney and liver function**

I try to oil pull a couple times a week, as my wife rolls her eyes at me. I've noticed fresher breath on the days I pull and a cleaner feeling in my mouth. I do believe oil pulling is effective at removing some harmful bacteria from the mouth and is a simple method to improve oral health.

Earthing (vitamin G)

One of the most important yet missing links to unleashing inner health is "vitamin G", or simply the ground! The earth is full of negatively charged ions and electrons, replenished continuously by the sun and lightning. Our bodies on the other hand are full of positive ions and electrons called free radicals. These free radical electrons bounce around the body damaging every tissue they run into and it takes antioxidants in our diet to reduce these damaging electrons. Without adequate antioxidant protection free radicals cause the damage that contributes to heart disease and cancer.

Modern research confirms that simply connecting to the earth can have a remarkable effect on our health. We were designed to be connected to planet Earth but modern times have disconnected us. We wear shoes made of insulating rubber, walk on pavement, and live and work in buildings with concrete floors. In other words, our bare skin rarely touches the ground.

It has been shown that when we connect our bare skin to the surface of the earth we are able to exchange energy. We can absorb the negative electrons from the ground and release the positive electrons building up in our bodies. This exchange of energy has been shown in studies (Ghaly and D. Teplitz, Journal of Alternative and Complementary Medicine) to benefit us in the following ways:

- **Reduce Inflammation & pain**
- **Strengthen the immune system**
- **Reduce heart disease**
- **Reduce the stress hormone cortisol**
- **Increase energy**
- **Improve mood**
- **Improve sleep**

Have you ever noticed that you feel good, have more energy, sleep better, and feel happier after spending time walking barefoot on the beach? There may be several factors at play here but certainly one of them is the connection to the earth's energy. I try to take my shoes off and connect to the earth as often as possible and have noticed a difference when I do. Patty no longer rolls her eyes at me for this one...she enjoys "earthing" now as well!

Tea Bag Rub

Most people know that tea, especially green tea, is very good for us. Tea is second to water as the most consumed drink in the world, and I believe it is also second to water as the healthiest drink in the world. Green tea has been consumed in Asia since the days of the Old Testament and Asian people are among the healthiest in the world. All tea whether green, black, oolong, or white come from the same plant but they are very different. Green tea goes through very little processing thus preserving the many antioxidants found in its leaves. Black tea, which is the most popular tea consumed in the United States, is allowed to oxidize in order to achieve a bolder, darker color and taste. This process reduces the amount of beneficial antioxidants.

Green tea contains very powerful antioxidants called polyphenols which are responsible for removing those damaging free radicals.

What is a Free Radical?

Free Radical (Noun): An especially reactive atom that has one or more unpaired electrons that can damage cells, proteins, and DNA by altering their chemical structure

— MERRIAM WEBSTER

Green tea consumption is associated with a reduced risk of heart disease by reducing the free radical damage to artery walls. Consumption of green tea may also reduce the risk of certain cancers, especially colon, bladder, stomach, and skin cancers. Green tea may also boost the immune system and it contains an amino acid called L-Theanine which is anti-anxiety and very relaxing.

It is well established that green tea has many health benefits but why does it make Patty roll her eyes at me? I have been drinking several cups of green tea every day for many years. On our second date, Patty and I decided to meet at a local coffee & tea joint and we sat outside enjoying our beverages, pleasant weather, and conversation. I of course got green tea and when the tea had finished steeping I removed the bag, squeezed the bag into the cup to ensure that I got as many polyphenols as possible, and wiped my face with the warm bag. Yes, I wiped my face with the warm tea bag right in front of this gorgeous lady whom I'm having a second date with! It only took a second to do and it was second nature to me, but it made a lasting impression on my date who still talks about it several years later. In fact, she texted her sister and wrote *"you'll never believe what this guy just did"*…and they laughed about it for weeks.

So, why did I wipe my face with the warm tea bag, almost ruining a chance at a 3rd date? While studying herbal medicine in Southern California, a professor of Chinese Medicine explained to us that the skin is the largest organ of the body and will absorb nutrients very easily. He recommended that we make a habit of absorbing extra antioxidants from the tea bag before discarding it by wiping our faces with it after steeping. I've been doing it ever since despite the eye rolling from Patty, and everyone around me when I do it in public. Plus, it's soothing and feels good!

Sniffing Frankincense

Frankincense was one of the gifts given to baby Jesus by the three kings. In those days, it was valued as highly as gold and held in high regard for thousands of years. It was known that frankincense had many healing properties, but it was also burned to purify the air, body, and soul. Modern research has identified that frankincense does have healing potential. Here are the uses of frankincense:

- **Asthma / Bronchial Infection / Shortness of Breath**
- **Cold / Flu / Nasal Congestion / Laryngitis**
- **Healthy Skin / Blemishes / Sores**
- **Arthritis / Joint Pain / Inflammation**

I utilize frankincense in many ways. I take boswellia, an Ayurvedic remedy for inflammation and pain internally in capsule form. Boswellia comes from frankincense. I also use frankincense in a steam diffuser when possible for the aromatherapy uses of the oil. Often though, I can be seen walking around the office with a bottle of frankincense oil up to my nose sniffing it. I have found this to be an excellent way to inhale the powerful, ancient healing properties of this gift of the Magi.

Conclusion

My wife Patty thinks I'm a nut but she willingly (for the most part) goes along with my recommendations about herbal remedies. I do tend to take things to the extreme at times but my passion for studying and teaching the 3000 year history of herbal medicine continues to get stronger. I may do some crazy, eye-rolling stuff but it's all based on solid research…or at least thousands of years of tradition. Look forward to driving your family members a little crazy as you *Unleash Your Inner Health!*

8

Traditional Chinese Medicine / Acupuncture / Thai Chi / Qigong

With Robert Bradley, LMBT, Thai Chi & Qigong instructor

I cannot write a book about the human body's desire for balance and health without discussing one of the oldest forms of healing known… TCM, or Traditional Chinese Medicine. It is important to know that over 4,000 years ago, Chinese healers knew more about how the body heals than many modern-day physicians. I have experienced and witnessed the healing of TCM and acupressure and believe in the healing power of Thai Chi and Qigong. Everything relates to the body's desire for balance and the power of the energy flow within us. I have studied Chinese herbal medicine but I am not an expert at the balancing and healing effects of acupuncture or Thai Chi.

So for this discussion I contacted my friend Robert Bradley, LMBT, Certified Sin Tien Wuji Thai Chi Qigong instructor. Robert has been studying TCM and acupuncture for many years and has a great understanding of the healing systems associated with them. He also practices and teaches Thai Chi and Qigong. Here's what Robert had to say about healing:

It seems to me that the body has the innate desire to achieve wellness in relation to its environment. Thus, there is always a balancing dance between the external and internal environments. For instance, a person who consistently exposes their head to the elements in winter may get a cold invasion and thus suffer from a head cold or an acute case of sinusitis. In this case the external environmental factor was "cold" and the internal environment did not have the fortitude to resist. Perhaps, it was the prolonged exposure to cold that wore down resistance or perhaps the internal environment was already weakened by other factors. The above example was a simplistic model; however, it does highlight a point. The point is that health may in a large part be dependent upon our bodies' ability to achieve auto-regulation in accordance to our external habitat. This balance between internal and external as well as balance itself is a huge conceptual Foundation of Acupuncture, Chinese Medicine, and Taichi/Qigong. This concept is captured in what many call the yin/yang symbol.

In my eyes, one cannot separate Chinese Medicine from the dao or "way". The "Way" can be described as living life in accordance with nature and what is natural. Living life downstream as opposed to upstream. Water doesn't flow up the mountain and neither should we. It creates problems. Water can't flow uphill because of gravity which is currently a law of nature. In fact, the sage phrase above outlines life in accordance with nature or balance. Humans live on the earth which moves around the sun, which moves the solar system that ebbs and flows with the movements of the galaxy, which moves according to the grander currents of the universe. Thus, as long as we eat with the seasons, dress for the seasons, and maintain seasonal practices maybe we can maintain some type of balance that equates to general wellbeing. In terms of longevity, it would be wise to go to bed earlier and wake up later in the winter because nature calls for us to do so.

Winter is related to water phase in Chinese Medicine. What happens to water when it is cold? It tends to slow down and consolidate, eventually forming ice if it is below freezing. If we shut out our distractions and cultivate our awareness we can notice that autumn makes us feel a little reclusive. There is less inclination to frolic and more inclination to gather inward like squirrels gathering nuts for the winter. We notice that even our thoughts tend to be more introspective. I definitely notice that I am in my head more in the winter. Truly, winter is a time to go within and do mental work on ourselves so that we may shed ideologies and mental/emotional traps that block us from our "true nature"; so we can be mentally and emotionally born anew in the spring. I often observe many people starting romantic relationships in the fall and suddenly falling out of love the following spring. They want to be tied down in the winter but not in the summer. We naturally desire to go out less in winter.

One concept of the "way" or dao is to view the human body as a microcosm of the macrocosmic whole. Imagine the ocean. When we think of this ecosystem we know it is teeming with life. Predators help with over population while plants and other organisms help to keep it clean. We all think of sharks as the top ocean predators. Well, if we think of a tide pool at low tide equipped with barnacles starfish, algae, crabs, and a few fish. Then the top predator of the tide pool may be the fish or crab. Nonetheless, this tide pool is a microcosm within the macrocosmic ocean. Surface ocean biology is driven by photosynthesis while deep ocean life is driven by chemosynthesis. Chemosynthesis is life based on methane coming out of deep hydrothermal vents in the ocean because sunlight cannot reach these deep ocean surfaces. Thus chemical exchange is what creates tube worms, crabs, and other organisms in this ecosystem. Methane acts as the sun of the deep. This again is a microcosm within a macrocosmic whole; however, in this example it is difficult to distinguish which is macro and which is micro. Cold deep ocean waters are recycled at the earth's poles into warm surface ocean waters. I mention the cycle of ocean water to demonstrate the observation of cycles in nature.

Early practitioners of Chinese medicine usually related nature to the body in this way. It is as if they viewed the body and nature in fractals. Thus, Chinese medicine sees physiology through a lens of cycles and phases much like seasons and other naturally occurring phenomena. The organs are grouped into pairs and these pairs are associated with phases of nature. These phases are water, wood, fire, earth, and metal. Water nourishes wood, wood builds fire and so on until we get to water again. Another way of looking at the phases is to imagine them as cycles of time. Wood is birth, fire is growth, earth is the climax, and metal is descent leading to water which is death. Or we can say wood is morning, fire is mid-morning, earth is noon, metal is afternoon and water is night. Then the cycle begins again with wood. It is the goal of the medicine to keep these phases balanced in accordance with each other. Wood cannot thrive if water is not abundant. For instance, the Liver and Gallbladder are grouped to form the wood phase; however, the wood phase is not just the liver and gallbladder. It is a continuum or frequency that resonates with a particular season and essence along with certain anatomical structures and physiological processes. The season is spring and therefore the wood phase is associated with renewal, birth, and sprouting forth. At this time it is worthy to mention that the liver is the only organ that can *regenerate* itself given it is not totally destroyed. The color associated with wood phase is green while the flavor is sour and the climatic factor associated with it is wind. Hence, in good health, the wood phase is responsible for a healthy breeze in the body and dictates movement. If one does not move enough or too much then problems can arise within the wood phase which can then cause problems with all the other phases.

I don't know if I mentioned it before but Classical Chinese Medicine is about cycles, phases, and balance of "qi". Okay, I didn't mention qi previously, so we will explore it now. Qi is usually described as life force or vital force much like prana in Ayruveda. Qi is not directly observed; however, you usually observe the manifestation of it. Actually qi is involved with everything in nature. Qi flows around the body as well as through the body and its internal organs. In classic texts, it is said that "the qi follows the blood". Thus, the movement of blood is a byproduct of the movement of qi. We know that blood moves in blood vessels. Arteries usher blood away from the heart carrying oxygen and nutrients to the tissues via capillaries while veins return deoxygenated blood back to the heart. Qi flows in an intricate channel system as well, known as the *jingluo*, which is a network of channels and collaterals that dictate the physiology of the body. The artist Alex Grey does a good job depicting the jingluo alongside the vascular system in many of his paintings of the human body. I often think of the jingluo as what many spiritualists call the ethereal body, one of the seven or five layers of a human being. The ethereal body is like a template that gives the framework for the physical body. It is in this sense that I would call Acupuncture an energetic medicine perhaps at the dismay of my colleagues who practice only western medicine. If the movement of qi in the jingluo corresponds with the movement of blood in the vascular system, then would it not be wise to proactively handle issues at the qi level before it turns into problems at the blood level? I like to think that the physical body is the last frontier in terms of energy. The ethereal body is one step up from this rock bottom dense material world. Problems such as cancer and other pathologies will show up in the jingluo and energetic body before they physically manifest. Thus, acupuncture and herbal medicine is truly a proactive medicine. The nutritive qi we gain from food and breathing allows us to create qi that circulates throughout our ethereal bodies building tissues and circulating fluids of the physical body.

Imagine a busy interstate equipped with exit ramps and side roads leading to main streets and avenues feeding a metropolitan. If there is traffic accident on the interstate, there could be blockages and delays that lead to more accidents which further congest the flow of the city traffic. This is what happens when there is a blockage of qi circulation in the jingluo. The jingluo or acupuncture channel system is a living network that circulates qi for many cycles night and day. Impedance of circulation leads to stagnation. Stagnation means lack of movement and buildup of excess. If a chronically injured muscle is ischemic (without blood) and full of fibrotic and scarred tissue, then that muscle has an accumulation of metabolic waste. Lack of blood means lack of movement and nutrients into to the tissue. Therefore, the muscle cannot get rid of the waste. The waste leads to diminished nerve response while neurotransmitter secretion becomes negatively altered. This is similar to what happens to qi. If we look at general low back pain, the sacrum and iliac crest are natural bony barriers separating the back from the gluteal muscles. This natural impedance usually combined with lack of movement easily leads to stagnation and pain in the lower back. This is usually called stagnation in the bladder channel which is the yang channel of the water phase. It is normal to be accompanied with some wood phase issues also in the hip. If we picture a beaver dam with a surplus of water on one side and less water on the opposite side and compare it to a qi obstruction, then one side has so much qi it is about to bust while the other side has so little qi it cannot support the surrounding environment. Acupuncture and Chinese Herbal Medicine seeks to balance these two sides by strengthening what is weak and reducing what is full for autonomous flow.

As mentioned previously stagnation and impedance are normally accompanied by lack of movement. Movement encourages venous return, lymph circulation, and, of course, qi circulation. Depending on the person, intense workouts can be too physically demanding and is not advised by many classical Chinese physicians because it is believed to put too much strain on the body. Furthermore, western science is now proving that intense exercise can cause rapid telomere shortening, which as we know leads to a decrease in life span.

"Tai Chi should be a dance your body recognizes even if you have never done it before"

Therefore, Tai Chi is perfect because it is vigorous enough to cause perspiration but gentle enough to float. Relaxation is crucial to the practice of Tai Chi. I always find myself feeling tension when I thought I was relaxed. So the work in Tai Chi is to achieve relaxation of the mind and the body. Tension leads to impedance of qi flow while chronic tension, that most of us carry, unknowingly leads to stagnation and inflammation. Inflammation and markers of it also lead to telomere shortening, qi stagnation, and pathologies. Tai Chi along with Acupuncture has been proven to relieve high blood pressure and curb diabetes significantly. Several studies have shown that Tai Chi builds more bone density than resistance training. Additionally there have been other studies that show how Tai Chi helps with Parkinson's disease. Consistent practice helps with balance, coordination, and cognition.

Qigong can be considered a predecessor to Tai Chi. There are probably are as many types of Qigong as there are people in the US. Maybe even more! Qi Gong translates to energy work and most Qi Gong involves breathing exercises to maximize an aspect of the nutritive qi that circulates throughout the body. Qi Gong works the jingluo pathways and seeks to open them allowing qi to flow all while guided by focused breathing.

I began looking for a Tai Chi/ Qi Gong teacher almost twenty years ago and found one by the name of Sifu David Chin. I found his system to be the best fit for me. The Sin Tien Wuji Qigong system he created includes two styles of Tai Chi, Yang and Original Yang (Quang Ping), and breathing exercises along with a unique set of Qi Gong that deeply cultivates awareness of both mind and body. I practice this system every day and personally feel its benefits. It is easy and I don't have to think too much. Thinking too much creates tension and that is not the goal. A lion does not have to think to be a lion. Tai Chi should be a dance your body recognizes even if you have never done it before.

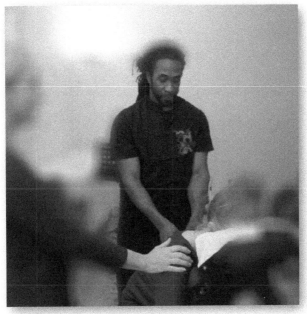

Robert Bradley

Action Plan: Seek out a licensed acupuncturist to keep you chi moving in the right direction...and unclog any stagnant chi. Find a Thai Chi or Qigong class or instructor and reap the benefits of exercise movements that are several thousand years old.

Resources

Many of the healing foods, teas, and herbs I discuss in this book are available at health food stores and grocery stores. For instance, you can easily find pure pomegranate juice and kombucha at most grocery stores while magnesium, curcumin, and beet root juice are all readily available at most community health food stores. But there are some things that are harder to find and some herbs that frankly I'm just very picky about the source. The following is a list of companies that I use personally, as well as in my practice, because I trust their quality and effectiveness:

Jiaogulan
Immortalitea
www.Immortalitea.com
Their jiaogulan is grown responsibly using all-organic farming methods, working directly with hill-tribe farmers in Northern Thailand. This is the only jiaogulan I drink and it tastes delicious. I enjoy a cup every morning and another after work.

Kava
Kava Root USA
www.KavaRootUSA.com
Their kava powder is imported directly from the birthplace of kava... Vanuatu. It is the kava that I have consumed nightly for over 10 years and instantly takes the edge off of my day!

Root of Happiness
www.RootOfHappiness.com
These guys know their kava! They source directly from the South Pacific Islands to provide kava to their two kava bar locations and online. In California, stop by the Root of Happiness Kava bar in Rancho

Cordova or Davis and enjoy a shell. They sell premium, quality, lab tested raw kava powders, extracts, tinctures, and more!

Cordyceps
Aloha Medicinals
www.AlohaMedicinals.com

This is the only cordyceps I consume. They grow their cordyceps in a low-oxygen, low temperature environment to mimic the climate of the Himalayan region where cordyceps grows in nature. This process makes their cordyceps the only true strain of cordyceps grown commercially. Visit their website for full details.

CBD Oil
West Coast CBD
www.WestCoastCBD.com

With popularity of CBD skyrocketing, I am always cautious about companies trying to jump on the bandwagon. Many companies do not have the expertise or quality that I look for. I trust CBD oil from these guys! It is top quality and contains what the label claims.

About Jeffrey Blair

Dr. Jeffrey Blair, PhD has been studying nutrition and herbal medicine for
over 25 years. He is Board Certified
by the AAMA and is a Fellow of The
Naturopathic Research Foundation.
He is the author of 4 books, Health: An
American Crisis, Dear God, Why Am I
So Tired?, Runology, and Unleash Your
Inner Health! He has been a guest on
radio and television shows around the
world and is a sought after speaker.
Dr. Blair has been a consultant to the
nutritional supplement industry for

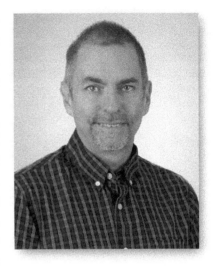

many years and has a passion for research and teaching. He is blessed
to have a wonderful wife, Patty...daughter Ashley...three step-daughters,
Lauren, Allison, and Molly...two dogs, Lucy and Mack...and a Bearded
Dragon lizard named Ricky! Dr. Blair is not afraid to take on the con-
troversial topics of the day including medical cannabis, the failures of
modern medicine, and failed diets! Dr. Blair is an avid hiker and competitive runner.

CPSIA information can be obtained
at www.ICGtesting.com
Printed in the USA
FFHW01n1134270718
47572366-51048FF

9 781545 321959